PRAISE FOR PHYSICIAN

"This deeply thoughtful book gives you a front row seat on a journey that will adjust your paradigm of the past, present, and future of medicine. Drawing from the fields of medicine, philosophy, physics, psychology, mathematics, and metaphysics, Kurapati creates a rich contextual tapestry around the evolution of the modern physician."

—Greg N. Korneluk, CEO,
International Council for Quality Care Inc. and author of
Physician Success Secrets: How the Best Get Better

"*Physician* by Dr. Rajeev Kurapati is a fascinating review of medical history. It explores the doctor-patient relationship but dives in deeper than typical writings on the subject to answer questions such as "Why me?" that patients may ask when suffering. Reading this book, it is easy to see how a patient or a healthcare worker can incorporate a higher thinking into addressing aspects of human suffering that are not normally addressed in the medical setting. I recommend this book to anyone who may ever need to see a doctor."

—Dr. Linda Girgis, Physician and author of
Inside Our Broken Healthcare System

"Dr. Kurapati beautifully weaves the lessons of history with personal stories, giving the reader a keen perspective of present-day medicine. *Physician* is very unique. It will bring the layperson and the professional to new grounds in understanding the evolving physician-patient relationship."

—Dr. Paul Ruggieri MD, FACS, Surgeon
and author of *The Cost of Cutting*

"Dr. Kurapati offers a fascinating review of the history of medicine that leads to an extraordinary vision for its future. Patients, families, and the entire healthcare team will all benefit!"

—Beth Boynton, RN, MS, and author of *Medical Improv:
A New Way to Teach Communication*

"Dr. Kurapati uses his book as an opportunity to delve into the evolution of medicine and the issues that have influenced us in the medical community over time. Art, science, emotion, religion, and technology all play a part in this informative book that encourages us to transform our practice of medicine and strengthen the physician-patient relationship."

—Dr. Jessica Willett, MD, Emergency physician and humanitarian

"As a hospice worker, I feel that this book is a must-read for anyone in the healthcare field. Dr. Kurapati understands and gives practical insight into the need for holistic healthcare."

—Kristy Matheson, LSW, Licensed social worker, hospice
and community educator, and public speaker

"*Physician* is an engaging, well-written account of how and why physicians should blend hard medical science with soft, thorough perspective. Dr. Kurapati details real patient experiences in part to explore the evolution of ancient history's view of medicine as well as to nudge current and budding physicians to be more eclectic."

—Elaine C. Pereira, MA, OTR/L CDC, CDP,
Occupational Therapist and author of *I Will Never Forget*

"The author gives an elegant account of how the roles of the typical physician have evolved over time with advancements in science and technology and how several societal forces have come to shape the doctor–patient relationship. The book is written in an engaging style and with minimal technical jargon; it is apt to enlighten not only health professionals but anybody interested in the history of the science and art of medicine, and in questions such as what it really means to be a physician, and what it means to provide patient-centered care."

—Dr. E. S. Prakash, MBBS

"Dr. Rajeev Kurapati's summary of medicine covers not only Western medicine, but the history of ancient China, India, and the Middle East, giving the reader a full understanding of how physicians went from spiritual and physical healers to the physical healers of today. He discusses how technology has affected and will continue to impact the physician–patient relationship going forward."

—Dr. Eiman Jahangir, MD, MPH, FACC, FAHA,
Cardiologist and clinical researcher

"Through his narrative, Dr. Kurapati sutures together the disparate aspects of medical care that have pervaded the ages. Kurapati waxes poetic in one moment, shifting to a clinical and succinct voice in the next, emulating the essence of medicine's evolution and bringing to bear the fact that medicine has wavered—at times struggled—between the poetic and sterile in its attempt to serve the patient. This book should leave the reader with a sense of possibility and personal reflection on what it means to be a healer-philosopher-educator."

—Jerome Stone, RN, Healthcare consultant, keynote speaker, and author of *Minding the Bedside*

"A stimulating account of how medicine advanced by getting physical."

—Kirkus Reviews

PHYSICIAN

HOW SCIENCE TRANSFORMED
the ART *of* MEDICINE

RAJEEV KURAPATI, MD

RIVER GROVE
BOOKS

This book is intended as a reference volume only. It is sold with the understanding that the publisher and author are not engaged in rendering any professional services. The information given here is designed to help you make informed decisions. If you suspect that you have a problem that might require professional treatment or advice, you should seek competent help. The names and identifying characteristics of persons referenced in this book, as well as identifying events and places, have been changed to protect the privacy of the individuals and their families.

Published by River Grove Books
Austin, TX
www.rivergrovebooks.com

Distributed by River Grove Books

Design and composition by Greenleaf Book Group
Cover design by Greenleaf Book Group
Cover image © Africa Studio, 2012. Used under license from Shutterstock.com

Cataloging-in-Publication data is available.

Print ISBN: 978-1-63299-145-4

eBook ISBN: 978-1-63299-146-1

First Edition

CONTENTS

For a long time, I wondered: Why is it that physicians and poets feel destined never to speak the same language? In other words, why is medical literature dry, devoid of rhyme and rhythm, and full of technical language, like an instruction manual describing the workings of a machine?

This book is the result of an earnest attempt to answer this seemingly simple question.

I have long felt that most of our confusion about *why* we do the things we do often clears up if we understand how we arrived here in the first place. A peek into the past is necessary in order to assemble the building blocks of how our culture designed our current version of the modern physician and what that means for patients today. So, I decided I would devote a portion of my life—three years, as it turns out—to absorbing walloping amounts of literature about medicine's past and pondering the future of healthcare. I reflected on the many patient encounters I've had over the years, picking out the ones that made an impact on me, both personally and professionally. The idea was to explore the depths of what it really means to be a doctor (and a patient) at this time in our human history.

As I threw myself into researching that initial question, I discovered many little-known aspects of the profession that were more than just intriguing; they seemed essential to the practice of medicine. It took me on a journey that revealed the fundamental assumptions that lay the foundation upon which modern medical science was built. It became a search for the meaning of *who I am as a physician* (as a person of science) within the context of my everyday experiences in the profession.

Society longed for a streamlined, regulated process that would make it easier and faster to receive medical care, but our existing healthcare climate leaves room for many questions of improvement. To name a few: How has the promise of medical technology influenced society's perception of death; How do physicians balance *thinking* with *feeling* when dealing with critically ill patients? Are we living in a technologically proficient but emotionally deficient medical landscape where doctors and patients feel like cogs in a relentless medical-industrial complex? And if this is the case, has it become our shared reality? Is it possible to overcome some of these *necessary* compromises we've had to absorb along the way? Most unnerving of all, as medical care becomes more and more digitized and automated, what value will the medical degree—a universal badge of respectability—continue to hold?

The book was structured in two parts. The first part tackles the historical narrative of how we arrived at the current version of medical science, the answer to my first question. The second part explores how this transformation of the healing tradition from a spiritual practice to a scientific one changed the very style and substance of how medicine is and will be practiced going forward.

I've approached this book with sensitivity to both patients and physicians. As part of this effort, I've avoided technical jargon and oversimplified some of the complicated scientific concepts. The names and identities of all patients and their families have been changed to preserve confidentiality with the exception of Father John Seiler, who granted permission to me to include our conversations in this book.

In writing this book, I aspired to uncover both the promise of modern medicine and its limitations. I hope that in reading this book you find new ways of looking at certain familiar ideas and deep-rooted perceptions. Perhaps you'll discover new ideas about your doctor, your patients, or even yourself.

I am indebted to my extraordinary patients from whom I learned as much as I did from my formal teachers, for instilling in me that medical practice is not simply diagnosing and treating an ailing body, but a competent and compassionate management of a vulnerable situation.

"WHY ME?"

The greatest mistake in the treatment of diseases is that there are physicians for
the body and physicians for the soul, although the two cannot be separated.

—PLATO

I'm running out of options, I thought to myself after the nurse, Sarah, paged me. She wanted to let me know that Trazodone—our fourth pill in a trial of treatments for our patient—also hadn't helped. I was becoming powerless to Walter's inability to have a restful night's sleep.

"He hardly slept again last night," Sarah explained, her voice flat.

"Is he still asking his questions?"

"Yup." She sighed at the other end of the phone. "I don't know what else to tell him."

"All right, thank you. I'll be in shortly." I hung up to plot the next steps of my treatment plan.

Our patient was Walter Stephenson, a 40-year-old African American man, though upon first glance he appeared older. Tall and moderately built, he looked rugged, with high cheekbones and a small gap between his two front teeth. His thick, curly hair was well kept, while his hands and abdomen were scattered with bruises from needle sticks, blown IV sites, and insulin injections.

Our staff knew him to be extremely pleasant, but over the course of his five-week stay, he'd grown agitated, lost weight, and stopped caring about his appearance.

Among his exhaustive list of ailments, insomnia was the most recent contender. Since I'd first admitted Walter to the general medical floor, four other specialists had joined me (his hospital physician) on his care team.

Making my way through the hospital during morning rounds, I walked into his room to the same view I'd seen for the last several days. He was lying in bed with his shirt off, flushed from the concoctions of IV medications he received around the clock. He stared blankly at the TV, giving his eyes a break every so often with an equally vacant gaze out the window. He no longer made direct eye contact with us—not out of indifference, but out of sheer inability to locate my eyes within the blur of his vision, a consequence of his near-blindness. Two framed pictures featuring his wife and son graced his nightstand. Alongside them were get-well cards and a handwritten note from his teenage son, which read, *Love you, Dad*. Walter's earbuds dangled along his neck and plugged into his iPhone, his most constant companion.

A distinct odor instantly repelled all who entered Walter's room— despite fastidious care, the smell of his rotting feet indicated an active infection. Because the mist burned his eyes and caused him to constantly sneeze, he didn't like for us to spray air freshener. The stench stuck to my clothes and in my nose for hours after I'd left his room, though it no longer seemed to bother Walter at all.

"Doc, can you please help me get some sleep?" The question was now part of our routine, a plea inching toward desperation as yet another sleepless night passed. The all-night vigils had become a type of confirmation of my patient's inability to thrive.

Eight years ago, then 32, Walter learned he had diabetes. Because he was adopted, he hadn't been aware of his potential risk factors. Blood work revealed severe kidney failure—the first of a series of utter disappointments regarding his health.

He was ordered to undergo dialysis three times a week for the rest of his life, which meant he was only able to work part time. Until two years ago, Walter had tried to live a relatively normal life, maintaining a steady job at a factory. As the disease progressed, however, his role was eventually limited to clerical duties for a short time until his near-blindness made it impossible for him to work altogether.

As the high sugar levels in his body damaged his nerves and blood vessels, he started losing vision in both of his eyes, and the sensation in his feet faded to a point where he couldn't feel the floor beneath him. It became easy to step on sharp objects without even noticing, and as a result, he developed dreaded diabetic foot ulcers, the type of wound that can silently chew up a leg.

The decline of his health had accelerated several weeks prior, after he developed an infection at the site of his dialysis catheter. The infection spread to the rest of his body and seeded his heart valves. Walter was put on IV antibiotics, but by then the other infection from his ulcerated foot had already spread to the bones in his toes. Little by little, surgeons removed parts of his feet to keep the infection from spreading. When he needed to get around the hospital, he utilized a wheelchair, though his activity had decreased drastically and had left him mostly bedridden.

While trying to make peace with the loss of his toes, Walter was hit with yet another setback when his entire foot had to be amputated due to the flesh-eating germs that were making a home in the bones of his legs. Unfortunately, even this couldn't eradicate the infection. Now, he was preparing for the biggest surgery of his life—leg amputation below the left knee.

He was up to 24 pills a day to manage his diabetes, kidney failure, anemia, nausea, insomnia, pain, and acid reflux, plus insulin injections and two IV antibiotics. Yes, he understood that with many medications there were uncomfortable side effects, but knowing this didn't necessarily make the reality any easier.

"I think you all feel that I'm supposed to be happy that I'm even alive," he groaned, helpless, agonizing during one of my visits. "You think that if I have to lose my foot, it's okay. But it's not okay, Doc."

When our conversations reached this point, I always made an effort to appease him the best I could. We'd recap his treatment plan—one he'd heard countless times—but still I offered the steps again each day as a matter of reassurance.

At some point, he'd always interrupt to ask, "Why is this happening to me?"

As a physician, my job is to explain the disease, treatment, and possible outcome in clear and understandable language. But by then, Walter thoroughly comprehended the medical explanation for his suffering. His question was more existential. What he wanted to know was "why is this happening to *me?*"

While Walter's question was valid, I needed to keep the conversation grounded in medicine. I did my best to direct him back to the treatment plan. "Let's get through the surgery and get rid of the infection in your foot. Things will get better," I said, knowing that despite our best efforts, things for Walter were never going to be the same.

As a medical professional, there are so many times when I feel like taking off my doctor's cap and fulfilling a more comforting role, and this was especially true with Walter. In certain moments, I wanted to sit down and explain that suffering is part of what makes us human, that we don't always have an answer to *why me*. A few times I even tried, but our discussion quickly turned into more of an idle lecture about the value of a supportive family and care team. My monologues felt unbearable even to me—these weren't the answers he was looking for, and we both knew that.

During the course of his hospital stay, Walter's once charming sense of humor slowly changed into nagging complaints. This was, understandably, an emotionally tumultuous period in his life. The visits from his friends and family grew fewer and shorter as his indifference wedged between his relationships—he was angry, mostly at himself.

Walter was being seen by a team of specialists, one for each affected part of his body: a cardiologist, a nephrologist, a surgeon, and an infection specialist. Individually, we tackled one area at a time, engrossed in his care while developing a treatment plan. Yet this frustrated Walter. "They just see the disease," he lamented, "not me as a person."

I realized that the amount of time and effort I spent listening wasn't really what concerned him. He wasn't even especially interested in my acknowledgment of his feelings about his condition. His frustration stemmed from only one thing, and that was my refusal to engage with or respond to his existential questions. He wanted me to discuss the meaning of his suffering. But, as a physician, I couldn't try to answer *why* he had to suffer in the first place.

Serious illness or loss often motivates us to seek answers to these big-picture struggles. But physicians are not trained, and frankly are not always willing, to devote much time pondering these *why me* sorts of inquiries with their patients. It isn't that doctors don't care enough about their patients to engage in this way, but it's a nearly universal adherence to the notion that, for a doctor, to heal the body means to accomplish something tangible: to clear out a clogged artery, to remove a tumor, to eradicate an infection, or to help an individual regain mobility. It's not part of a physician's routine to heal metaphysical distress by addressing existential questions like *Why is this happening to me? Is there a purpose behind this suffering?*

When the current team couldn't ease Walter's emotional distress, the next addition was a psychiatrist. The psychiatrist, after a thorough evaluation, signed off stating that Walter suffered from situational depression due to his compounding medical conditions and advised that we increase the dose of the antidepressants he was taking. The psychiatrist's firm recommendation was that we continue to improve Walter's general health in order to improve his mood. Still, despite the help from the psychiatrist, days continued to pass with no results. At that point, we'd officially run out of specialists to help uplift our disheartened patient.

. . .

As humans, we're the only species that can contemplate our mortality. This ability is exactly what makes us the dominant species on Earth. What we passionately glorify as human progress is the result of our desperation for self-preservation. This obsession alone has resulted in some of our greatest achievements in medicine and technology. But the ability to reflect upon and be motivated by our mortality comes at a price. When an illness becomes a constant reminder of our death, we perpetually live in the shadow of our own apocalypse. In the case of Walter Stephenson, it was the impending dissolution of his leg. He saw us—his caretakers—as missionaries bent on spreading bad news.

Walter had every reason to be terrified of his situation. It's human nature to wish for a peaceful death after a long and well-lived life. Of course, the number of times this wish is fulfilled are few and far between. For some, death comes sooner than we'd like, and that's perhaps the very reason to fear it. But with advances in medical treatments, death can now be deferred for days, weeks, months, or even years, a blessing that brings fears of its own: disability, dependency, and pain. Walter was experiencing all of this at the same time—a fear of dying at a young age and a fear of living in his current state of pain and dependency.

The sickbed became a dark and lonely place. Walter seemed to have come to the conclusion that we, as physicians, were simply prolonging his death with all of these surgeries, tests, and medications. We tried switching Walter to different antidepressants, but these also didn't really make a difference in his mood. None of our interventions could pacify his emotional distress. And how could they?

All along, what we were really doing was attempting to fit his symptoms into certain diagnostic pigeonholes. In Walter's case, based on his symptoms, we fit him effortlessly into the diagnostic criteria of depression based on his lack of interest, hopelessness, and insomnia, for which standardized counseling and medications are customary recommendations.

But Walter kept saying, "Doc, I'm not depressed. I'm looking for answers." The very act of him asking such perplexing questions compelled us to view him as even more "depressed." The more he persisted in this state, the stronger his severity of depression was, according to customary diagnostic norms.

When faced with imminent loss, few people can pretend that they're without fear, but most of us hopelessly yearn for answers to the question of *why me*? No medication can give the right answer, because this is not a mental illness. This isn't an ailment to be cured with medications—it is our earnest, helpless plea to understand why we suffer. When Walter was tormented by the thought of *what did I do to deserve this*?, our medical theories failed him.

Rather than simply letting Walter continue on with these deep questions unanswered, there was one person who we thought might successfully address his questions head on—the hospital chaplain. That's when Father John Seiler joined our care team.

Our goal as doctors was to make Walter better, both physically and emotionally. If his current state continued, Walter was at risk of withdrawing completely and refusing his treatments, at which point saving his life would become next to impossible. We had high hopes that Father John, as we called him, could engage in Walter's existential rhetoric, appease his need for sympathetic dialogue, and help him internalize his suffering, thus easing his emotional distress.

A week passed. I started to notice a slight change in Walter's attitude. For once, he stopped asking me the difficult question of *why me*? He seemed to be more agreeable to the relatively severe treatment plans we were proposing: the amputation, more antibiotics, and a longer hospital stay. He wasn't without moments of melancholy and he still struggled with sleep, but there were glimpses of improvement. A great sense of relief washed over me on the morning Walter said, "Doc, I'll work with you to get me through this."

He became characteristically more accepting of our recommendations. Our treatment plan didn't change at all, but his attitude toward it did. With this gradual shift in Walter's perspective, I sought out Father John to ask what he was doing to help Walter.

I ran into the chaplain a few days later as he was exiting Walter's room. I asked if he had a moment to discuss our common patient. It's unusual for physicians to interact with the chaplains, especially regarding patients, but he certainly must have noticed the buzz of enthusiasm lighting my face. "How about tomorrow morning?" he suggested. I agreed as he limped away, leaning heavily on his walker as he made his way down the hall.

The next morning, I arrived at Father John's office, right next to the small chapel of our hospital. When I entered, I found him sitting in a chair in front of a study table in a rather small room, slightly larger than a cubicle. He offered me the seat across from his. Father John, in his black clerical attire, had a welcoming way about him, with a pleasant face, thin build, and Zen-like voice. "How can I help you?" he asked, and I could tell that this was exactly how he began every conversation.

After introducing myself one more time, I responded, "We share a patient, Walter."

"Oh, Walter Stephenson." Father John's face fell. He rubbed his cheeks with his palms and shook his head. "Terrible. Too much happening too fast for him. He's only 40," he sighed. By the expression on his face, it was as though he'd absorbed some of the man's own suffering.

"Very sad," I agreed. Then I cleared my throat and started by asking what he did on a daily basis with Walter.

"For all patients," he explained, "I perform what Catholics call the sacrament of anointing of the sick. We pray that their anxieties are eased, that their sickness be healed, that their fears turn to hope." Father John talked as if he had all the time in the world, though I knew he didn't; like me, he had to "round" on several patients that morning.

"But what do you actually *do* to the patient?" I asked like a curious child.

"I place my hands on Walter's head and anoint his forehead with the oil that's been blessed during the week. This is part of my daily routine with everyone I see." He stopped somewhat abruptly, confident he'd told me everything I needed to know.

But I needed more. I needed to know how Walter's inquiries were answered from the Father's perspective: Why was he suffering? "How did you approach Walter's questions?" I pressed.

Without wavering, Father John replied, "The Bible teaches us that we all have sinned and fall short of the glory of God. Pain and suffering are not right; they are the tragic consequences of living in a fallen world." It was clear he'd given this answer to many patients over many years.

This is the expected response, I thought. For those who are believers, it can explain why we suffer, although when severe illness strikes, even the most devout believers struggle to make peace.

"Despite your prayers," I asked, "what do you tell patients when they don't get better? What if the infection consumes Walter, and he dies soon?" I didn't want to come across as abrasive, but I did want to at least attempt to bring us closer to the root of my curiosity. "What do you say to explain how religion can justify suffering? For instance, why do babies get sick?"

He paused for a moment. "We don't know the answer to everything, but there's one thing we know for sure." Then he quoted directly from the Bible: "'We are to comfort one another with the knowledge that our destiny is secure in the arms of the Lord, even in the face of suffering and death.' In other words, suffering is not to be perceived as our apocalypse."

I kept my posture neutral but continued to press. "But Walter doesn't deserve this. Is it not unfair?"

In his usual unwavering demeanor, he said something significant, something no doctor I know would ever utter to their patients: "Healing can occur without cure."

Now it was my turn to pause as I tried to get this right. I felt almost anxious as I spoke. "So, if Walter loses his limbs or, worse, say he even dies, he's still healed?"

"Correct. Healing could mean cure of illness, yes. But it could also be found in death." His voice was soft yet affirming. "All of this—both great joy and great suffering—is part of His plan. Through suffering, something profound is revealed to us. It is something magnificent, something unique for each one of us."

It's fascinating how charged some words can become, I thought.

"And talking about loss of limbs," Father John said as he straightened his back, gazing straight into my eyes and exhaling deeply, "look at me." He directed my attention to his left pant leg as he lifted it to show me a prosthetic metal limb, which replaced his entire appendage from the hip down. It made sense to me then why his pant leg was covered in holes—marks from where the metal had rubbed through the cloth. I felt grateful to be in the presence of this 81-year-old man who limped his way around the hospital comforting the sick and the dying. Those next few seconds felt especially long to me.

He pointed toward his walker, "That's been my constant companion." He went on to detail that, following knee-replacement surgery, a stubborn circulation problem had grown progressively worse, subsequently robbing him of his leg. "What can you do?" he shrugged, as if he'd described an every-day misfortune, not the loss of an entire limb. "I still feel blessed to have lived the life I've had. I was raised to be a compassionate and caring person, and I'm eternally thankful to God for that," he said, delicately patting his prosthetic. It was apparent that this wasn't a role he'd simply chosen from the stack of identities modern society offered.

I could have stayed and picked his brain all morning. Instead, after he patiently answered a few more of my pointed questions, I closed my meeting with Father John by asking what he personally thought about Walter's situation.

"Walter has his good days and bad days, but overall he seems a little better." He worried that Walter might spiral down and withdraw further if he wasn't well supported. This was Father John's daily quest—to offer a sense of comfort and help patients regain their willingness to fight. Then, pointing his palms toward me, he told me that as a doctor I am also *His* instrument in healing people.

Father John was trying, and to an extent succeeding, in something we as medical professionals were struggling to do. He was able to regain a better connection with Walter, as well as with his family and friends, as a critical element in the success of his care. The chaplain persuaded Walter's family to spend more time with him and to reestablish a sense of community he so desperately needed.

When people come to visit, this breaks the isolation of being hospital-bound and reaffirms the patient's significance and their human connection, providing tangible comfort. When serious illness robs us of our ability to gain perspective in life, visits from spiritual individuals like Father John can provide a larger-than-life presence and reinvigorate our sense of hope.

I couldn't tell if Walter, with his failing health, was ever going to be able to truly come to terms with his situation. What was obvious, though, was his ability to better cooperate with his medical team, giving him a far better chance to recover some of his health.

. . .

One thing has stuck with me since my encounter with Father John: **Healing can occur without a cure.** Initially, I had difficulty wrapping my head around this. I had to step out of my role of doctor to truly understand what it meant. For a physician, healing means curing an illness, the eradication of disease, and the establishment of physical health. When a doctor says, "You're healed of cancer," they literally mean that you are physically cured of it, at least temporarily.

But Father John was looking at healing from another dimension. Among dozens of religions, hundreds of denominations, and thousands of sects, each one thinks it alone holds the key to true healing. Despite their differences, what's common among all spiritual traditions is the way each strives to provide a sense of meaning and explain why bad things happen.

Physicians interact with patients during some of the most crucial moments of their lives—at their births and on their deathbeds, when they're sickest or when they've experienced substantial recovery—events loaded with existential significance. Despite this, physicians usually don't bring their personal beliefs into the discussion. As caring as physicians can be, we are also people of science, meaning that doctors strive to stay within the boundaries of scientific reasoning. Some fear that ineffable concepts such as the soul and spirit can quickly drift the discussion into a metaphysical fog.

I have had a few instances in which patients have asked me to pray for them before going into a procedure. My usual answer is, "I certainly will," with ease. My version of prayer, though, doesn't include verbal expression, religious services, or rituals. It simply means an earnest appeal to something greater than myself for the benefit of the sick. Yet when I've asked my fellow doctors what they do when patients ask them to pray, the general consensus has been that they most often regard the exercise as one that falls outside of their role. One colleague even said, "To actually pray? Oh. It would be uncomfortable, wouldn't it?"

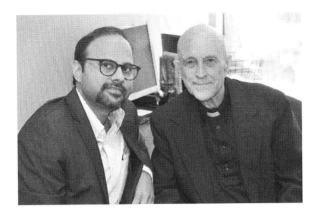

Rajeev Kurapati and Father John Seiler (1934–2016)—
December 28, 2015, in his office at Ft. Thomas Hospital, Kentucky

The distinction is clear. Physicians are healers of the body and priests are healers of the soul, for those who believe one exists.

As I was pondering my discussion with Father John, an undeniable reality dawned upon me. Weren't the physicians of our antiquity also priests and philosophers? I reflected on how odd it would be to serve as a physician and a priest at the same time. But this was how medicine was practiced for the better part of history all over the world. Priest-physicians served as healers of both the body and the soul. As I meditated on this thought, I decided to dig more deeply into this former practice.

Evidently, the root meaning of the word "clergy" is *a learned person*, which is also the root for "clever." Well into the eighteenth century, clergy were also physicians, mathematicians, and astronomers. What transformed the priest—the healer of antiquity—into a person of science? What transformed medicine into, as some say, a soulless profession? How was the modern doctor made?

PART ONE

THE PRIEST-PHYSICIAN

"Religion and medicine originally shared a common orientation—both *holiness* and *healing* are words adopted from a common Latin origin meaning *that which must be preserved intact*. Such concepts ensured unity of medicine and faith— physician-priest-philosopher—the curer of bodies and the healer of souls."

. . .

"As long as the human body was viewed as the 'divine temple,' doctors could not cut, probe, or maim our mortal parts in the way required for adequate study. If only this spiritual element could be separated from the physician, perhaps there would be a chance to unravel the mysteries. But how?"

CHAPTER 1

THE NATURAL PHILOSOPHER

Fourteenth-century men seemed to have regarded their doctor in rather
the same way as twentieth-century men are apt to regard their priest.

—PHILIP ZIEGLER, *THE BLACK DEATH*

The philosophies of one age have become the absurdities of the next, and
the foolishness of yesterday has become the wisdom of tomorrow.

—SIR WILLIAM OSLER

As a modern doctor, I understand that I have no explanation for some
diseases. Why, for example, do kids suffer from cancer? When a mother
grieves as she watches her child succumb to a slow death from leukemia,
what can I tell her?

As a physician who practices within the limits of science, the best
reason I can offer is what scientific medicine provides. To the distressed
parent, the mortality statistics may come across as a dispassionate rundown of clinical realities. I might say that perhaps the leukemia is the
result of an inherited genetic mutation, passed on unwittingly from parent to child. But this explanation doesn't do anything to ease the guilt

that a parent feels when a child is incurably ill. I can give nothing to this mother to console her sorrow-laden heart.

A similar explanation applies to many cancers in adults, particularly when these cancer-causing mutations are exacerbated by lifestyle and environmental causes such as smoking, exposure to chemicals, or too much time in the sun. But for kids, little is known about the causes of these mutations.

Yes, cancer can be caused by tobacco smoke or by an inherited trait, but research finds that most of the mutations leading to cancer crop up naturally. Every time a perfectly normal cell divides, it makes several mistakes when it copies its DNA. These are naturally occurring mutations. Most of the time, those mutations are located in unimportant parts of DNA. That's good luck. But occasionally they occur in a cancer-provoking gene. That's bad luck.

After two or three of these troublemaker genes get mutated in the same cell, they can transform that healthy cell into a cancerous one. What we know so far is that about two-thirds of the total mutations are random, slightly less than a third are due to the environment, and only five percent are hereditary—numbers that vary depending on the type of cancer. Lung cancer, for instance, is largely the result of environmental causes, while the vast majority of childhood cancer is a result of these bad-luck mutations. Of course, people can reduce their risk of preventable cancer by avoiding tobacco, eating well, and maintaining a healthy body weight, but the reality is still that most mutations arise naturally— we have no control over them.

Parents often think that, somehow, they're responsible for their child's cancer, but in actuality these cancers would have occurred no matter what. Even if we do narrow down what causes these genetic aberrations in children, we still fall short of explaining why kids *have* to suffer from these often fatal illnesses in the first place.

We might also ask why the immune system sometimes attacks our own tissues to cause rheumatoid arthritis, diabetes, lupus, or multiple sclerosis.

On the night she was diagnosed with celiac disease, a young woman in her early thirties lamented:

> Tonight was the night of a nervous breakdown, a crying fest. I have never felt such a burden in all of my life. . . . I met with the gastroenterologist today, had MORE blood work to confirm there are no other diseases at play with the celiac disease. I was asked to seek a nutritionist. I was also encouraged to find a support group for those with celiac disease . . . and then spent an overwhelming amount of time buying stuff I can eat. It finally sunk in today that this will be the norm for the entirety of my life, and [I] cried of frustration trying to explain everything the doctor told me to my husband who is looking at me like I am crazy. I am scared of all the changes . . . changes that could mean a healthy wife or days of sickness if we don't do things the right way. . . .

Where modern medicine fails to find causes of certain illnesses, evolutionary theories try to fill the gap. Consider the painful condition gout. The best available explanation of why individuals are afflicted with gout is based around the evolutionary theory that humans and great apes have higher blood uric acid levels due to a specific genetic mutation that occurred about 15 million years ago. Uric acid, as an antioxidant, protects against aging and cancer. Logically, natural selection probably led to higher uric acid levels in the blood of our ancestors because protection against cancer and the ailing consequences of senescence are especially useful in a species that lives as long as we do.

English physician Thomas Sydenham, describing how a person with gout spends a restless night in *A Treatise of the Gout and Dropsy* in 1683, writes:

The patient goes to bed, and sleeps quietly, till about two in the morning, when he is awakened by a severe pain. The pain resembles that of a dislocated bone . . . [and] becomes so exquisitely painful, as not to endure the weight of the clothes, nor the shaking of the room from a person's walking briskly therein.

Sydenham wrote with such clarity because he suffered terribly from gout himself. Even the evolutionary explanation of a disease, as logical as it may sound, doesn't pacify the individual's longing to know why they have to suffer.

In its current state, modern medicine remains ill equipped to answer the patient's questions, *Why me? Why specifically me? Why should I suffer?*

I'm trained to address, from a particular viewpoint based on scientific medicine, how the body works and why some people get certain diseases when others don't. Take strokes, for example. Uncontrolled high blood pressure, the consumption of fatty foods that raise cholesterol, and genes predisposed to atherosclerosis are major causes. But medical science, in its current state, struggles to explain why one individual over another succumbs to a stroke in the first place—why the self-correcting mechanisms of the body fail.

When faced with life-threatening illnesses like cancer, doctors are left to guide patients through a sea of uncertainty. Cancer is complicated, and it's difficult to compare one type or one particular stage to another. Compounding cancer's many consequences, many patients are also frustrated and scared, while family members frequently feel sad, guilty, and helpless. However hard doctors may attempt to coach a patient through this trying time, our efforts often fall short, failing to lend meaningful emotional satisfaction.

The scientific approach is bound by what we can perceive with evidence. Doctors are no different. When asked by a patient, *Why did I suffer from a stroke*, the answer might be, *Because of uncontrolled blood pressure.*

And after running few tests, a doctor's response to *Well, why do I have high blood pressure?* could be, *It likely runs in your family.*

Why does it run in my family?

Perhaps there's an evolutionary explanation.

Beyond a point, this line of *Why me?* questioning turns into a metaphysical preoccupation. Such philosophical pursuit is beyond the limits of scientific reason and is thus deemed outside the scope of a doctor's role. The decisions of a scientifically trained physician are driven by facts, not by what he or she happens to believe. When the conversation trails past the boundary of objective proof, the true answers to these questions become unsatisfying to patients: *We don't know.*

Scientists aggressively pursue the *why* of many things, although there's a limit to how far down the rabbit hole they're willing to go. When science, in all of its glory, can't explain why we have to suffer from an illness, patients become emotionally exhausted and inwardly defeated.

This is why the most difficult discussion physicians have with patients and their families doesn't involve laying out a detailed vignette of tests or procedures to diagnose an illness, or explaining a complicated surgery. In fact, most doctors find these exercises intellectually stimulating and professionally fulfilling. Instead, the most demanding conversation occurs when a doctor can't find the root of a sickness—when, despite their best efforts, medical professionals are left stumped. Perhaps even more challenging is determining what to say if all treatments fail. The life-altering, and in some cases life-ending, decisions made by patients and their families may literally hinge on the choice of words the doctor uses when delivering this news.

If a patient is admitted to the hospital with no meaningful recovery from terminal illness, a rookie physician might start by asking the patient's family, "What would you like us to do if your mother's heart stops beating or she stops breathing? Do you want us to do everything we possibly can?"

Most family members would, of course, instantly reply, "YES, do everything you can to keep my mother alive," when what they'd actually mean to say was, "Do everything you can to keep my mother *comfortable*."

After several years of grooming, physicians come to more fully realize the power behind the words they choose, learning how to steer patients and families toward truly digesting the impact of their decisions. Instead of using the phrase "do everything," a physician might delicately elaborate: "We could press on her chest, which could result in cracking her ribs, shock her heart, insert a breathing tube down her throat to put her on an artificial ventilator, or. . . ." Usually this approach garners a much different response from the earlier knee-jerk reactions a physician might have elicited. In these instances, patients and families tend to listen intently as the seasoned physician offers an alternative: "If your mother decides she doesn't desire these aggressive, life-prolonging measures, we can let nature take its course."

When there's nothing left to be done by medical science, physicians may attempt to offer varying levels of comfort to grieving families. Still, most take meticulous care not to use phrases like "let God decide" or "the patient will be in a better place." No scientifically trained modern physician explicitly invokes supernatural forces in their treatment plans or deliberately uses the terms *spirit* or *soul* in their discussions. To ward off sickness, our medical education trains us to rely only on the abundance of medical knowledge at our disposal. Rather than illnesses being predetermined by any supernatural force, we know that our fates and the fates of our patients are determined by our genes, environments, lifestyles, habits, and decisions.

For the ancient medicine man, though, supernatural forces played the most deterministic role in patients' fates. The village healer of antiquity underwent tedious training to attain certain mystical powers. The medicine man would retire in isolation to "make medicine," that is, to learn the art of healing. Here, he'd fast, pray, and surcharge himself with intense penance or other occult practices to the point of ecstasy. In this state, he'd receive word from the gods through some phenomenon of nature to guide his future.

When he returned to the tribe, he would use his newfound "powers" to cure maladies. One popular belief of pre-medieval times was that illness involved losing part of our soul, so restoration was a key component of healing. The medicine man would enter into a trance to travel to the spiritual world, where he'd then be able to retrieve the soul of the ailing person and return it to them.

Essentially, illness was seen as a sort of personal consequence. Using his mystical powers, the medicine man would first strive to pin down which affliction visited the victim and caused the illness. It was usually a curse or a possession that took the blame. The village healer then warded off the affliction using his occult powers. In modern medical linguistics, we see the relics of this terminology when we regard illness as an invader and our bodies as a battlefield with the use of phrases like "attacked by disease" or "fighting off infection."

The visible, traumatic injuries were treated far more practically (and far more successfully) with bandages, stitches, or splints. When it came to non-traumatic internal ailments, however, our ancients had no clue.

The ancient Egyptians, for example, laid down a systematic method to deal with traumatic injuries. This method was meticulously inscribed in the oldest known surviving medical text, the Edwin Smith Papyrus, dating about 1600 BC.

The physicians classified injuries based on diagnoses they made by finger exploration, then followed a logical treatment plan. They even predicted the outcome of an injury based on the symptoms with surprisingly impressive accuracy. Each case was classified by one of three different verdicts: (1) favorable, (2) uncertain, or (3) unfavorable. A gaping wound in the head penetrating to the bone would be classified as "an ailment which I will treat." Whereas, for a wound penetrating to the bone and splitting the skull with the addition of fever and stiffness (of the neck), the classification shifted to "ailment will not be treated" surgically.

Knowledge of anatomy, the palpable aspect of our biology, was garnered largely by the observation of grievously wounded soldiers and animal dissections. Conversely, diseases that presented without apparent physical trauma were more likely to be diagnosed as being brought about by malevolent spirits or demons. In this case, it seemed like a logical part of the healing process for ancient physicians to invoke the deities of protection.

Primitive people firmly believed disease was sent by the gods as a punishment for moral transgressions, delivered either to the transgressor or to a loved one or confidant. They also didn't believe that sickness struck randomly. Disease was an act of retribution—deception, disloyalty, or theft might explain why someone was sick. With their supernatural beliefs, the medicine man had made-up theories for every aliment under the sun.

Healers often stumbled when attempting to cure diseases, but always played a necessary and important role in offering comfort. In that sense, ancient physicians were able to better perform their duties in this one aspect of care. Since ancient times through modern day, this remains the primary goal of a healer, as observed in 1800 by Dr. Edward Trudeau, founder of a tuberculosis sanatorium: "To cure sometimes, to relieve often, to comfort always."

Because healing was regarded as the outcome of personal, social, and religious beliefs in ancient society, treatment was not merely achieved through the use of therapeutics. Illness was a vital concern for the whole community—a collective suffering. It required rituals that ceremonially cleansed the polluted, offered reparations, and warded off ghosts. Rituals, incantations, and sacrifices were thus essential to this process, as were faith and therapeutics.

Many religions around the world maintain that illness is a manifestation of sin or misdeeds, and ardent followers of these religions continue to believe in such convictions to this day. To most modern doctors, however, disease is recognized as a biological phenomenon concerning only the individual who's suffering.

The result is that suffering can be a lonely fight of one individual against an unknown adversary, a solitary battle in an unchartered territory. When we suffer a stroke or succumb to cancer, physicians don't place blame on or attribute this to a moral trespass or the result of sin. This is true even for doctors who believe there are factors contributing to illnesses beyond the boundaries of human comprehension.

For a doctor like me, there's no room in modern medicine for concepts such as the soul or spirit in curing illnesses. This, however, is a radical departure from how it all started.

. . .

Religion and medicine originally shared a common orientation—both *holiness* and *healing* are words adopted from a common Latin origin meaning *that which must be preserved intact.* Such concepts ensured unity of medicine and faith—physician-priest-philosopher—the curer of bodies and the healer of souls. The delineations between the body, mind, and soul were nonexistent for our forbearers. In Greek philosophy, the righteous mind was a direct reflection of the heavens, and all learning was the path to spiritual fulfillment.

Most physicians in ancient times were temple priests who *knew* the reasons why things happened in nature, particularly to humanity. Mythological tales of gods and super-humans filled in many of the gaps: Sickness was a consequence of angering the gods, and no one dared to challenge that notion. Appeasing the gods was a way to cope with uncertainties and provided a seemingly convincing path to health and prosperity.

Yet even then, mythology as an "explain all" caused dissonance for some who sought rational interpretations of all phenomena rather than attribution to supernatural theories. One such push back in ancient Greece arose 600 years before the Christian era, during which creations of human intellect achieved lasting glory. For the first time in the history of Western civilization, people began looking here on Earth rather than toward the heavens for answers to the *why* of all things.

One prevailing belief was that we are a synthesis of both the mortal body and the immortal soul. Greek philosopher Plato theorized that death applies only to our flesh, while the soul survives unharmed. The soul was seen as the supreme commander of all human functions, a concept detailed by Plato's prized student Aristotle in his "first-cause" principle. Essentially this principle suggests that there is something on which all else is predicated but which isn't predicated on anything else. In the case of humans, the soul is the first cause of all phenomena. According to Aristotle, the soul controlled all vital functions of organic life: vegetative, sensory, and intellect.

Originally, concepts of the soul and the mind frequently overlapped to describe the metaphysical dimension of our body. In fact, the word *soul*, derived from its Greek root *psukhe*—which later became *psyche*— was related to breath (*pneuma*). A dead person was thought to have lost his *psyche* by the release of the soul from the body.

In the transition from the belief that everything could be attributed solely to the gods to the idea that nature controlled the *why* of things, the meaning of God and nature frequently merged. By the sixth century BC, philosophers began to distance the gods from earthly phenomena by describing them as supernatural beings that occupied the heavens, far removed from humankind. This separation furthered when they began identifying earthly elements as life forces, a concept based on their observations of natural phenomena.

Because these individuals were interested in the study of nature, the term that evolved to describe them was "natural philosophers." A natural philosopher was generally a multifaceted individual, being a physician, philosopher, theologian, mathematician, metaphysician, social reformer, and counsel to the rulers all in one.

The most differentiated and highly specialized natural philosopher of ancient times would be equivalent to a scientist in present day. One such natural philosopher was the Greek philosopher and priest Thales, who earned his place in history three centuries before Aristotle. His theory was rooted in simple logic: All things in nature need water to live. Life on Earth hinged on the presence of water. Evaporation was proof that all things of water eventually return to the universe from which they came. Thales concluded water to be the alpha and omega of all things, breaking the traditions of existing mythology to which most philosophers later followed suit.

That's not to say that religion became irrelevant. On the contrary, gods became even more powerful. The emblem "Rx," which is still used by physicians, was originally the symbol representing the eye of the god Horus, an Egyptian symbol of protection. It was first used as an invocation on prescriptions by Babylonian physicians.

The introduction of the gods as heavenly rather than earthly deities led to a transformation in Greek beliefs. Gods who had once been half-man, half-beast were finally separated from their animalistic tendencies and became symbols of perfection. The question of human imperfection, however, remained. Answering this very question was the preoccupation of the medicine man.

Pythagoras, the successor of Thales, had a different take on natural phenomena. Unlike the organic conception of this topic by his predecessors, Pythagoras was convinced the universe was defined by numbers. He likened bodily functions to a finely tuned musical instrument. Like musical scales, which are based on a series of numerical opposites, he believed that a well-balanced human body required the maintenance of opposites as well. Although he differed from his predecessors theoretically, he advocated that maintaining health occurred through the balance of four humors. By this time, the great physicians of the era agreed upon the firmly established humoral theory of healing.

Using the humoral theory to explain health and disease was simple and easy for both healers and patients. As such, this model of describing the workings of the human body has stuck with us for nearly 23 centuries.

The human body was thought to contain a mix of these four humors (in this context, meaning *fluids*): black bile, yellow or red bile, blood, and phlegm. Blood as the life-giving fluid became the most significant of the four humors because it provided nourishment to the body. When disordered, however, it caused inflammation and fever. This is why the term "blood poisoning" for sepsis is still in use.

Each individual possessed a particular humoral makeup, and an imbalance of these was believed to result in deposition of noxious substances, leading to diseases and death. Practitioners therefore used therapeutic techniques that imitated the body's natural healing mechanisms to balance these humors. Treatments consisted of assisted expulsion of poisons through the usual excretory organs using cathartics and enemas to increase bowel moments, expectorants to induce coughing, and diuretics to induce urination. The most relied-upon technique was bloodletting, which included cutting open veins in selected parts of the body to bleed the patient of "excess" blood. These treatments "purged" the patient of bad humors. Techniques capable of accomplishing balance of more than one humor were called *panaceas* or cure-all, and bloodletting was the most popular. Other less common avenues were massaging, irritating the skin by inducing sores, and burning the skin to extract the offending poisons from the vicinity of internal organs.

In the process of developing this approach to healing, new terminology was introduced. *Eucrasia* was the term given to the proper mix of all four humors, while *dyscrasia* denoted imbalance. The relics of this humoral theory still linger in most modern medical linguistics. Current-day physicians like me commonly use the word "blood dyscrasias" to indicate pathological disorders such as leukemia or hemophilia, in which the constituents of the blood are abnormal or are present in abnormal quantity.

It was Pythagoras's student Empedocles who later introduced the idea of the four elements of fire, air, earth, and water into the equation. Inspired by his teacher, Empedocles believed four to be the magic number of the universe; everything within it was comprised of four elements: Blood, being the life force, represented air; phlegm, being cold and wet, represented water; yellow or red bile, aiding in burning the food, represented fire; and black bile, maintaining body nutrients, represented earth.

During this time, medicine was a restless market comprised of competing healers: incantatory priests, exorcists, sorcerers, fortune tellers, and witch doctors. In this medical bazaar, each seller could pitch his or her wares, in opposition to or in cooperation with others, and the choice was left to the patient.

It was Hippocrates who changed the fate of this medical marketplace by emphasizing that clinical medicine is a discipline based on the practical application of intelligent analysis. Today, this is common knowledge among doctors, but when Hippocrates purportedly said, "It is the sick man who matters, not man's theory of sickness," the thought was revolutionary.

Hippocrates, born into a family of priest-physician lineage around 460 BC, popularized the nascent humoral theory and expanded it further. He evaluated health in terms of fluid balance, which included not only diseases but mental attitudes as well. Blood represented extroverted and social temperaments; yellow and red bile represented people with energy, passion, and charisma; phlegm represented dependability and affection; and black bile represented creativity, kindness, and consideration. Like the elements attached to them, the temperaments were viewed as complementary opposites. Successors continued to work the nascent humoral theory into a convincing body of knowledge that was passed on to generations of healers.

. . .

As priest-physicians, our ancient healers were convinced that together, the concept of the soul as the supreme commander of all activities *and* the theory of the four humors provided the best answers to *why* diseases occurred. When the humors were out of balance, it was impossible for the mind, body, and soul to be at ease. Medical practitioners developed corresponding cures to address these imbalances. Practices like witchcraft, magic, and incantation were used to heal the spirit, while bloodletting, typically with leeches or sharp instruments, was the preferred treatment to balance humors. Practitioners and patients adhered to these methods with fierce conviction because such practices assured the promise of balancing the spirit and body—the only gateway to healing.

However, Hippocrates did not see medicine as a superstitious practice. To him, the priest was separate from the physician, and proper understanding of disease required direct observation and evaluation, not faith. He cast aside the idea of disease being some sort of supernatural possession as ludicrous. Hippocrates understood that there was a very clear line between what was thought to be demonic possession and epilepsy, and that purifications and incantations were not satisfactory treatments of the latter. "Magic" was considered pointless, for he believed that nature was the true healer of disease, and thus he relied on a simple philosophy of not interfering too much. He felt that not only was disease caused by nature, it was also healed by nature in a process of bringing everything back into balance.

Although Hippocrates drew a distinct line between myth and medicine, he did not renounce the power of the gods. In fact, he readily acknowledged the limitations of medicine. When charged with heresy, he expressed his obedience: "Before the gods, the physicians bow, since they have no superabundance of power in their art." From his humility grew the Hippocratic Oath.

The oath, sworn under the gods, once began with:

> I swear by Apollo, and Asklepios and Hygieia and Panaceia and all the gods and goddesses, making them my witness, that I will fulfill according to my ability and judgment this oath and this covenant.

Though it has undergone many changes since it was first introduced, the oath is still taken by doctors today. Hippocrates was faithful to tradition in assigning "a grand place to nature" as the decisive healer. He dutifully believed not only that the "physician is only nature's assistant," but also limited the role of the gods.

According to his pupils, Hippocrates was the first physician who attempted to separate medicine from philosophy. Before him, the learned physicians of ancient Greece like Pythagoras, Demokritos, and Thales were far more dedicated to being philosophers. Hippocrates felt that they were more interested in developing philosophical theories than in healing the sick. He wrote:

> It is impossible to understand medicine without knowing what man is, how he first appeared, and how he in the beginning became a being. . . . As for me, I believe that all the speeches of sophists . . . and all that they have written about nature, belong rather to the business of writing than to medicine itself.

Hippocrates sought to free medicine from philosophy, but he did not succeed. Philosophy continued to regard medicine under its confines, and the medicine man refused to give up philosophical speculation.

Hippocrates's vision of separating physician from philosopher was inter-rupted by the path laid by an individual who single-handedly influenced how medicine was practiced for centuries. His name was Galen.

CHAPTER 2

INTELLECTUAL HIBERNATION

> A physician who fails to enter the body of a patient with the
> lamp of knowledge and understanding can never treat disease. He
> should first study all the factors, including environment, which
> influences a patient's disease, then prescribe treatment.
>
> —CHARAKA

More than 400 years after Hippocrates, Roman Emperor Marcus Aurelius declared, "Rome has but one physician—Galen." He was given the
title Clarissius by his followers, meaning *the most brilliant*. Galen's work
led to a vast encyclopedia of medicine, comprising 12 volumes that each
averaged more than 1,000 pages but was thought to represent less than
a third of his complete writings. So extensive was his work that the surviving texts amounted to nearly half of all the literature from ancient
Greece. During the Medieval Era, Galen was quoted and praised even
more than Hippocrates.

Despite his impact on medicine, no medical student or physician of
our time would likely know anything about him or his theories unless
they happened to develop a passion for medical history. Educated in

the epicenter of Greek education, the School of Alexandria, Galen went on to be all but forgotten, an outlier among his fellow alumni—Euclid, Archimedes, and Ptolemy—who were glorified throughout history books. By the nineteenth century, the medical community began to diminish Galen's legacy and eventually discard it entirely from medical literature. This wasn't due to any shortcomings of Galen himself, however. In fact, it was quite the opposite. The immensity of his personality and ingenuity dominated the medical establishment to such a degree that it gave birth to a rigid dogmatism that ultimately stifled medical advancement for centuries.

As the physician to the gladiators of the High Priest of Asia and one of the most influential men of his time, Galen claimed that the High Priest chose him over other doctors after he disemboweled an ape and then challenged other physicians to repair the damage. When none of them could, Galen performed the surgery himself, sealing his reputation as the "chosen one." His predecessors saw 60 gladiator deaths during their tenure, while when Galen held the title there were only 5, reinforcing his brilliance.

To Hippocrates's prevailing humoral theory, Galen added the layer of seasons, associating each with a humoral element: blood and air with spring, yellow or red bile and fire with summer, black bile and earth with autumn, and water and phlegm with winter. He believed that each person possessed a unique and specific balance of the four elements.

Galen's other contributions included a theory that the role of the arterial system was to spread *pneuma* from the lungs throughout the body. This particular concept was actually an impressively close approximation to what we know today, given that oxygen wasn't discovered for several hundred more years.

However, there were also many concepts for which Galen missed the mark, such as a collection of incorrect assumptions about human physiology. He erroneously believed that the circulatory system was comprised of two separate, one-way distribution channels rather than a single unified system. He also inaccurately theorized that blood was manufactured in the liver and carried by the veins to nourish tissues— being absorbed and depleted, not circulated, along the way.

While Galen emphasized the necessity of observation for understanding medicine, he also believed that every aspect of the human body harbored an indwelling spirit. He observed that "Every man who looks at things with an open mind, seeing a spirit living in this mass of flesh and humors, and examining the structure of any animal whatever . . . will comprehend the excellence of spirit which is in heaven."

The physician in him made numerous contributions to medical understanding, while the philosopher in him built a foundation of rigid doctrines that hindered further medical progress for centuries after his death.

Galen took philosophical theories from academic circles and established them firmly into medical practice. Inspired by Aristotle's theory of the soul, Galen proposed his own version. At the time, Aristotle's 400-year-old theory was popular among philosophical circles and academia. Aristotle suggested that the soul, as the inner ethereal aspect of each person, has three distinct elements: the appetite (or the desire), the spirited, and the mental or rational.

Galen furthered this theory by assigning parts of the soul to different parts of the body—the rational to the brain, the spirited to the heart, and the appetite to the liver. Balance of the soul was of equal importance to balance of the body. A person burdened with uncontrollable emotions, for instance, was thought to have too much blood and was "high spirited." The role of physicians was to re-establish perfect health by balancing the humors and the soul.

Where Hippocrates tried to disentangle the physician from the philosopher, Galen strengthened the relationship and spread the concept of a unified role throughout much of the Western world via his treatise

That the Best Physician Is also a Philosopher. Though Galen was a strong admirer of Hippocrates to the extent that he referred to the practice of medicine as "Hippocrates' Art," the Hippocratic vision of separating the physician from philosopher did not materialize until Galen's teachings were overturned centuries later. Galen wrote that "In order to discover the nature of the body, and the distinctions between disease, and the indications for remedies . . . philosophy is necessary for physicians if they are to use the Art [of medicine] correctly."

In the centuries after Galen, the West went through major social and cultural transformations. Greece was lost to the rise of the Roman Empire, and after Rome's collapse in the fourth and fifth centuries, Western civilization lurked in the shadow of the empire's past glory. This was a time when the future seemed more horrid than the past. As Christianity swept through the West, scholars turned to ancients like Aristotle, whose contributions were cemented in cultural history. The Aristotelian view of the universe was so closely tied to proof of God's existence that questioning the Aristotelian doctrine amounted to questioning divinity itself.

Aristotle's theories were so undisputed they were still being practiced sixteen centuries later. By this time, Aristotle's philosophy was blended with Christian theology and ethics, forming a conceptual framework that remained unquestioned throughout the remainder of the Middle Ages. It was so influential that any new philosophical idea of the time was impelled to fit within the scope of the Aristotelian system of thought.

Medieval natural philosophers, looking for the purposes underlying various natural phenomena, considered questions relating to God, the human soul, and ethics to be of the highest significance. The human body was considered the "high point" of God's creation; thus, when a person died, their body was considered sacred. Because of this, funeral rites were thought to be a critical component of a successful afterlife. The concept of resurrection was also widely accepted. The pathway to salvation rested on the righteous belief that we are saved through faith. Because of such beliefs, human dissections were strictly prohibited.

The Catholic Church didn't end the prohibition of public dissection at universities until the early 1300s. The knowledge of anatomy was acquired mostly through the study and observation of the external appearance of the body, as well as from the bodies of animals that were slaughtered for food or killed for sacrifice in religious ceremonies. Until the fourteenth century, dissection was illegal unless the body belonged to a criminal who was delivered to anatomists from prisons by royal sanction.

With the ban on dissection lifted, anatomists finally gained full reign to study the human form. Despite this, the practice of surgery maintained a lower reputation than that of other medical practices for a long time. The tradition dates back to several centuries before the time of Moses, when laws were written that regulated surgeons' practice. The Code of Hammurabi, composed some 4,000 years ago, is one example of an elaborate codification of laws. It stated that "If a surgeon operates on a man for a severe wound and causes the man's death; or opens an abscess [in the eye] of a man and destroys the man's eye, they shall cut off his fingers."

Such laws resulted in dissections being performed by surgical assistants, called "barbers," while professors lectured from a safe distance, one step removed from responsibility or blame. Meanwhile, non-surgeon physicians remained exempt from any failure to diagnose or cure an illness. They belonged to the priestly class and did not fall within the same scope of regulations. Because the popular belief among priest-physicians was that the gods sent down disease, a person in this role, by certain signs, foretold the future course of an illness. This conviction had a lasting impression on the practice of medicine, and religion and healing were left closely associated. Medical knowledge was bent within the framework of a closely woven synthesis of theology and philosophy.

. . .

By the fourteenth century, many aspects of human intellect had advanced, including the arts, architecture, mathematics, astronomy, and politics. The aspects of human endeavor that didn't fit within the master plan formulated by the thinkers of the church, on the other hand, didn't fare quite as well. The study of medicine was one of these, and it suffered greatly. In the fifteenth century, the Swiss philosopher and physician Paracelsus, who is credited with founding the discipline of Toxicology, defined four pillars of medicine: philosophy, astrology, alchemy, and virtue. Paracelsus discussed the will of God upon the health of man, noting that "The physician is the servant of nature and God is the master of nature." Philosophy and theology each continued to be joined hand-in-hand with medicine.

While bodily functions were explained through numerous theories, we didn't yet have a clue about the mechanisms by which various drugs and herbs acted upon the body when they were used to treat ailments. Up until this time, processes within the human body had been based merely on speculation, largely through the lasting lens of Galen's humoral theory.

Even hundreds of years later, Galen's teachings prevailed as the last word in medicine. The books of medical students were filled with exclamations of wonder at the "wisdom of the Creator who created all the parts with a purpose so obvious to Galen." As late as the 1600s, to earn a diploma for Doctor of Medicine, students were required to recite an oath that included this line: "Fellows must never speak disrespectfully of Galen."

Galen's theories became the foundation of authority of all medical writers and physicians, resulting in the establishment of a medical orthodoxy that went undisputed. Questioning Galen was tantamount to doubting the wisdom of the Greek lineage all the way back to Plato,

Aristotle, Pythagoras, and Hippocrates. Physicians didn't just learn from Galen, they worshiped his teachings as infallible notions with unshakable trust. Medicine, as science, couldn't progress until the world discarded Galen's theories. Yet, no one dared to question his doctrines.

As religion and philosophy came to influence every aspect of the human endeavor, in particular with regard to its stronghold in medicine, advancements in the understanding of health and disease came to a standstill. Scientific study was pursued only in a quest to understand God, and man's role in His vast creation. The human body was held as a vessel of God, a masterpiece of His creation. Cathedral schools maintained the monopoly on medical learning and education, where, under the supervision of the bishops, youth were instructed and prepared for admission to medical education only after taking holy orders in the church.

. . .

While Western Europe was held tightly in the grasp of the Catholic Church, a major revolution was born in the Arabian Peninsula of Western Asia: the rise and spread of Islam. In AD 622, Muhammad fought for his life with a small band of devoted followers and fled to a small city called *Yathrib* (later known as Medina). Filled with passion for Muhammad's zeal and his teachings, the Arabs were able to spread the newfound religion to half of the then-known world by the next century. For this population, scriptures served not only as spiritual guidance, but also as instruction manuals for healing traditions.

For physicians, this required a delicate act of attempting to synthesize reason with revelation. Drawing from the database of knowledge provided by Greek, Persian, and Hindu texts, Islamic scholars developed an interesting combination of philosophy and medicine. Galen and Hippocrates made a particularly heavy impact on them—the humoral theory survived for centuries through Arabic translations. The Islamic scholars also compiled many Greek and Roman texts into encyclopedias, beginning in the ninth century and lasting well into the nineteenth. This was the first civilization to systematically catalogue knowledge gathered from different continents on a massive scale.

Arabs and Persians were strongly influenced by existing theories, and while they had valuable opportunities to unravel the mysteries of human biology, they struggled to advance their medical knowledge as a result of the iron hand of religion. In tandem with the grasp of Christianity, the rise of Islam in other parts of the world brought additional restrictions on medicine.

This made the practical study of anatomy and physiology nearly impossible, resulting in medical knowledge that was based on observation and inferences rather than direct experimentation. Ibn as-Nafi, an Arabic physician during the 1200s, was the first to crack the understanding of pulmonary blood circulation and gas exchange. As time went on, though, he refused human dissections because of his strong belief in the religious teachings that condemned the act. Even with such barriers to intellectual growth, Islamic healers didn't simply build on the ideas laid forth by Greek medicine; Arabic physicians were able to make many original innovations in spite of such restrictions. It's interesting to envision what may have been for these curiously tenacious thinkers had these barriers from dogma been removed.

Even during the darkest times of intellectual hibernation, there were occasional glimmers of hope, but not much came to fruition. For instance, a precious opportunity to advance the understanding of human physiology came in the form of a genius child prodigy named Ibn Sina, born in Persia in AD 980. At a young age, Sina studied theology, philosophy, and science, gradually developing an interest in medicine. Credited as one of the original thinkers of experimental medicine, he detailed his theories in *The Canon of Medicine*, one of the many books he wrote during his lifetime.

Ibn Sina[1] brought attention to a glaring issue in medicine, arguing that "Just because a drug is given to a patient and the patient recovers, it can't simply be assumed that the drug was the cure." He argued that every technique and drug must be methodically tested in a controlled environment, void of as many variables as possible. While this certainly was a precursor for the scientific method, Sina was highly influenced by theology, having memorized the Qur'an by age 10. Despite his promotion of methodical study, he was firmly against dissecting animals and forbade human experiments.

Under these circumstances, there was essentially no way to learn human physiology since animals were not to be tested due to religious and ethical reasons. These original ideas promising great intellectual potential were either blatantly dismissed or veered into a blind alley due to theological preoccupations. Progress was stymied in this part of the world as well.

. . .

Aristotle's most famous student, Alexander the Great, helped spread the doctrines of his teacher to the East through his unprecedented conquests, before his untimely death in 323 BC. Though Aristotelian doctrines reached most of the known world at the time, the Greek philosophy never took hold in India and South East Asia. Most of the changes occurring in the West were limited to this region until European colonization in the seventeenth century.

The millennia-old indigenous Ayurveda healing method resembled

---

1 This spark of intellectual creativity should be put in context, though, as a true rarity of its time. Persians, descendants of ancient Mesopotamia, had an extraordinarily creative culture noted for their original works in philosophy, literature, art, and architecture, at least until Arab conquests wiped out their indigenous religion. The Arabs coerced the Persians to convert to Islam, which essentially brought an end to their ingenuity. Ibn Sina, a descendant of Zoroastrian faith, was therefore born Muslim.

the humoral theory of the Greeks, though it emerged independently. All ancient philosophers, both from the East and the West, saw the human body as a microcosm, or a *tiny universe*, that reflected a macrocosm, the *large universe*. The fundamental premise was that the inner environment, enclosed by a bag of skin within the human body, was a reflection of nature. Even the root word for "physiology," *physi*, literally means *nature*.

The ancients long held the belief that nature is a balance of the elements—air, fire, earth, and water. To the natural philosopher, this balance of elements was perfectly reflected within the human body. The Hindu philosophers divided human nature (pertaining to both mind and body) into three major categories, each influenced by three energies. An elaborate swath of knowledge was synthesized by associating different energies with different bodily functions and mental attitudes. The *Vata* (air or wind), *Pitta* (heat or fire), and *Kapha* (water or fluid) were thought to govern specific bodily functions and corresponding mentalities. For instance, Pitta was associated with digestion and metabolism. Any imbalance in this energy lead to dysfunction, including both heartburn and related behavioral disturbances, such as argumentative and short-tempered behavioral disturbances.

Like diagnosis, treatment also involved every aspect of a patient's life. Factors included vitality, the season, digestive power, age, state of mind, habits, diet, natural stage of disease, and more. After gauging these elements, a medication was selected. Most of the time, healers would prepare herbal medications individually, each one adapted to the specific needs of the patient. This approach to health and disease was meticulously practiced and passed on to successive generations.

In present day, Ayurveda is seen as a pseudoscience—more superstition than true clinical practice. Its current perception has been reduced mostly to herbs and oils, with practitioners touting its safety over other modern medical practices due to a less-heavy reliance on synthetically manufactured drugs. For centuries, however, it was this medical practice that safe-guarded one of the world's oldest civilizations.

Though India has faced many epidemics since the eighteenth century, no major pandemic was ever recorded before this, lending credence to ancient healing and hygiene practices. The Black Death, for instance, a plague that originated in central Asia in the fourteenth century, killed about 40 percent of Egypt's population and half of Paris's. Florence lost more than 60,000 citizens, and Hamburg and Bremen saw 60 percent perish—all due to a single disease. The effect was so powerful that from the fourteenth century, the recovery period was called the Renaissance—literally meaning *rebirth*—from the devastation of the plague (although it also refers to the birth of individuals with unquenchable curiosity). About a third of Europe died before authorities even had time to determine the origin, which was traced to Asia. Despite this, Hindus somehow fortified themselves against the wrath of this great plague even while the rest of the world was swept away by its devastation. In fact, it was discovered that the Indian subcontinent may have been the only area of Eurasia to have population growth during the fourteenth century.

Perhaps Ayurvedic practitioners realized the importance of preventative and supportive care long before anyone else. Or perhaps they were extremely lucky, which is hard to fathom considering how an entire civilization survived against some of the worst plagues in history.

In ancient times, medical knowledge in India was passed on through oral transmission of the Vedas, the sacred Hindu texts. The principles of Ayurveda were brought into prominence and further developed by the three greatest names in Hindu medicine: Susruta, Charaka, and Vaghbata.

Life for Hindus is seen as *maya*, the transient illusion of an unchanging Brahman (the creative God principle), which caused histories and biographies to be looked upon as the embodiment of flimsy vanities. The dates of historic milestones were, therefore, not accurately preserved.

The *Sushruta Samhita*, whose authorship is ascribed to Susruta, an ancient Hindu physician and surgeon who lived sometime between 700 and 600 BC, devised detailed teaching techniques and modules for practicing surgery. Skills for incision and excisions were acquired through practice on vegetables or mud-filled leather bags, scraping on animal skins, or puncturing veins of dead animals and lotus stalks. This dedicated practical curriculum made ancient Indians more accomplished in anatomy than their contemporaries elsewhere.

Over time, the authors of these healing theories became the ultimate authority because they represented originality. These authentic thinkers developed elaborate healing practices based on their keen observation in order to understand health and disease. Because every aspect of life was intimately linked to their spiritual philosophies, these therapeutics were deemed sacred, written by great physicians in poetic and literary richness. Constrained by their utmost reverence, successors were hesitant to tinker with these original texts and ideas. Obedience was institutionalized. Challenging or even critiquing ancient theories was condemned because of the moral implications, and as a result the understanding of human biology did not change much beyond what had already been theorized centuries earlier.

The healers of the ancient tradition thus became victims of their own brilliance.

· · ·

Just like the ancient Hindus, the Chinese also had their own theories regarding bodily functions and illness that were tightly linked to their philosophical interpretation of nature. Despite cultural isolation, China was largely influenced by India as Buddhism made its way into the country. Yoga, Ayurveda, and knowledge from other cultures also filtered into China by the Chinese ambassador Zhang Qian as a result of his travels to Mesopotamia, Syria, and Egypt.

The idea of energy flow being responsible for all life, the common theme throughout all of ancient medicine, prevailed in China for thousands of years. Synonymous to the Indian concept of *Prana*, or life force, in China the *Chi* referred to the energy that permeates all life. The Chi is believed to flow through the body in channels called meridians, each of which is influenced by a specific organ. Wellness is the result of a balanced flow of Chi through the body. If the flow of energy is blocked, we experience illness and pain as a result. The goal of physicians was ultimately to get the patient back to a state of equilibrium by balancing the Chi.

Inserting thin needles into selected points in these meridians was believed to allow energy to flow again, thus balancing the Chi so the body could repair itself to optimal health. This was the basis of acupuncture, which is still practiced today.

In ancient China, unlike other medical communities, medical knowledge was revered as a sort of secret power. Each doctor kept his techniques to himself, passing them on only to a son or, sometimes, a mentee in an uninterrupted line.

China is responsible for many firsts in medicine. Emperor Huang Ti (2650 BC) was credited with discovering circulation of the blood more than 4,000 years before William Harvey. The Chinese were able to inoculate against smallpox by blowing dried pustule crusts up the nose hundreds of years before Edward Jenner's discovery in late-eighteenth-century England.

Hua Tuo, born in AD 190, was one of the greatest Chinese surgeons. Surgeon to the King of Wei, he was able to remove a gangrenous spleen in a patient using an elixir of effervescing powder in wine to produce an anesthetic. Tuo also went against the grain of his contemporaries as a strong advocate of systematic physical examination, though he continued to practice acupuncture on a few regions of the body.

During the seventh and eighth centuries, Chinese medical doctrines spread across the world. Arabic and Indian missionaries of Islam and Buddhism were not only influenced by China, but also directly influenced Chinese culture as well. Since their missions necessitated the translation of Sanskrit and Arabic writings into Chinese and vice versa, medical knowledge was passed back and forth. This resulted in a hodgepodge of a healing system, combining aspects of various practices.

Much like how the West had halted its own forward progress through the idolization of Galen and Aristotle, the East too caged themselves in the shadow of their past glory for centuries. In explaining *why* an individual succumbs to illness, the people of ancient times also relied heavily on many artisanal practices such as numerology, palm reading, and even dream analysis. Instead of inquiring about knowledge based on hard facts, metaphysical and pagan traditions arose and became astoundingly lucrative.

Every culture all over the world was swarmed with cult-like theories that were firmly established as gospels of truth, which severely limited advancement in our understanding of human biology. The frame of reference became fixed, and the body of knowledge remained non-negotiable.

Physicians, for instance, didn't know why people were dying of fevers until the sixteenth century. Causes of fever were ascribed to everything from the gods to bad air, hence *mal-aria*. It took the devastating plagues of the Middle Ages before practitioners began to think that perhaps something solid must transmit disease from one person to another.

The medieval Italian physician Girolamo Fracastoro hypothesized that epidemics progressed via unseen seeds that swiftly propagated. He theorized they were spread by breath or air, by drinking from the same cup as or lying with an unkempt lover, by clothes, combs, coins, or anything infected. In short, he was the first to describe the mechanism of the spread of infections as we know it today, but he lacked a means to test his theory. The human operating system remained a mystery.

Centuries passed. Still, no one had a clue about how to translate the language of the human biology and unravel its many functions—from how the body regulates its own internal milieu to how it senses changes from outside its boundary to restore balance, and why those fool-proof mechanisms sometimes fail.

The story of medicine is mostly the story of the fallibility of our knowledge about ourselves, largely because for so long we could not conceptually conceive a method to test new ideas and to validate accepted wisdom. To really understand the mysteries of the human body, an entirely new way of thinking was required. We persisted in our own follies for too long.

As long as the human body was viewed as the "divine temple," doctors could not cut, probe, or maim our mortal parts in the way required for adequate study. If only this spiritual element could be separated from the physician, perhaps there would be a chance to unravel the mysteries. But how? Healers needed a method that would be accepted universally and would prohibit political and religious intervention—a method that would be systematized across all knowledge so that no one would question its validity. The medical community had already endured centuries of intellectual hibernation. It was high time to reinvent our methods.

CHAPTER 3

BREAKING THE IRON MOLD

> Tradition is the presentness of the past.
>
> —T.S. ELIOT

> I profess to learn and to teach anatomy not from books but from dissections, not from the tenets of Philosophers but from the fabric of Nature.
>
> —WILLIAM HARVEY

High priests and local residents reverently gathered around the coffin in the cathedral in Frombrok, Northern Poland, on Saturday May 22, 2010. The mortal remains of a man were blessed with holy water by some of Poland's highest-ranking clerics before an honor guard ceremoniously carried the coffin through the streets of the country for all of the community to see. Following the procession, the remains were buried again, nearly 500 years after the body had been laid to rest in an unmarked grave.

This was no ordinary man. He was, as they say, the man who put the "sun at the center of our universe." These were the remains of a person who, out of his sheer interest in astronomy, dedicated more than three

decades to crunching complex mathematical calculations in his free time
to develop a theory that would forever change our place in the cosmos.
Once a canon and doctor at a Polish church, this man single-handedly
ignited the modern scientific spirit. This man was Nicolaus Copernicus.

Ironically, this sixteenth-century priest-physician, mathematician,
and astronomer was far from idolized at the time of his death. When
he was buried beneath the floor of the cathedral in Frombrok, the exact
location of his unmarked grave was left unknown.

At the urging of a local bishop, scientists began searching in 2004
for the astronomer's remains. Eventually, the search team turned up the
remains of a 70-year-old man—the age Copernicus was when he died.
DNA analysis from the teeth and bones matched that of hairs found
in one of his books, leading scientists to conclude that they had finally
found Copernicus. To right a wrong committed nearly half a millennia
earlier, the church provided Copernicus with a proper burial, finally
lauding him as a hero.

The archbishop, along with the highest church authorities of the
deeply Catholic country, praised Copernicus for "his hard work, devotion, and above all, his scientific genius." This adoration was a stark
contrast to the way his work was perceived after his lifetime, when his
theories were condemned by the Catholic Church as heretical.

Immediately after its publication, the book was withdrawn from
circulation and was added to the church's list of prohibited writings,
pending "corrections." Nine sentences that represented the heliocentric
system were to be omitted before the book was formally approved for
publication again.

Anticipating such a backlash on his theories, Copernicus took meticulous care before his ideas became public. He ingeniously dedicated the
first copy of his book to Pope Paul III, whom Copernicus asked to protect him from vilification. In the dedication, he wrote:

Perhaps there will be babblers who claim to be judges of astronomy although completely ignorant of the subject and, badly distorting some passages of Scripture to their purpose, will dare to find fault with my undertaking and censure it. Hence scholars need not be surprised if any such person will likewise ridicule me.

Copernicus lived in the time when freedom of thought was heavily constrained by tradition, authority, and established belief. He was one of the first to tactfully challenge those restraints, which led the way for others to do the same. He received the first printed copy of his book *On the Revolutions of the Celestial Spheres* just hours before he took his last breath in 1543. It was in this same year that another groundbreaking book took shape as well: *On the Fabric of the Human Body* by a young anatomist named Andreas Vesalius. Together these two works sparked a radical change in our worldview. Ironically, the revolution in our thinking about both our external universe and the inner world beneath our skin occurred at the exact same time, and both gained momentum in the century that followed.

Unlike the soft-spoken, introverted, and relatively unknown Copernicus, Vesalius was outspoken, unbridled, and regarded as a prodigy of his time. The day after he received his doctorate, Vesalius was offered the position of Chair of Surgery and Anatomy at Italy's University of Padua.

Vesalius grew in notoriety as the top anatomist of his generation as he debunked glaring errors in the assumptions of Galen. Contrary to what Galen had preached, Vesalius discovered the human jaw was made up of a single bone, not two, and that the breast bone was only three, not seven.

In the course of Vesalius's meticulous dissections on human corpses stolen from the gallows, he made a striking discovery: Galen had relied on the dissection of apes and incorrectly attributed some of his anatomical findings of these animals to the human body. Vesalius set to work dissecting an animal cadaver and a human cadaver simultaneously as a means of demonstrating the anatomical differences and thus uncovering errors in Galen's theories.

Disgruntled with how anatomy was taught in universities, Vesalius once commented that "less is offered to the student than a butcher in a stall could teach the doctor." He went on to identify some 200 of Galen's errors, declaring boldly to his students that "everyone will be able to see it for himself" in the dissected human cadaver.

For the first time in history, the 1,500-year authority Galen once held was challenged by supported proof. Before Vesalius, anatomy had only been described in prose without illustrations. Vesalius exposed the inaccuracies of his predecessors by composing a book, bound in tanned human skin, in which he used impressive line drawings to communicate correct human anatomy. To create these anatomically correct images, Vesalius looked to the young artist Johann Stephan van Calcar, who also deeply understood the body. It wasn't unique for artists of this era to become experts on the human form—Donatello, Raphael, Verrocchio, and other famous artists were part of an unbroken line of truly great creative talents who mastered this skill. The final product, *On the Fabric of the Human Body*, was comprised of 663 pages and included 300 elaborate illustrations. Vesalius presented the first published copy of this magnus opus bound in silk of imperial purple, with specially hand-painted illustrations not found in any other copy, to the then Holy Roman Emperor Charles V. Vesalius, who was 28 at the time, spent his entire wealth and dedicated all of his efforts to the success of the book.

Apart from challenging the anatomical constructs of Galen, he even steered clear of addressing the theories of prominent ancient Greek philosophers. In Vesalius's own words: "To avoid running afoul of some idle talker here, or some critic of doctrine, I shall completely avoid this dispute concerning the types of soul and their location . . . and about the opinions of Plato, Aristotle, Galen, or their interpreters." He freed himself from the traditional methods of thinking that were emblematic of the Renaissance—a radical departure from his predecessors.

Though the long era of Galen's ideological grasp was weakened when his errors were brought to light in publications like those by Vesalius, this wasn't without resistance. Despite clear proof of his accuracy, Vesalius was ignored and shamed after he announced his discoveries, as the majority of physicians still considered Galen's work to be "most perfect and complete." This belief was so ingrained that some even considered Vesalius's work blasphemous. Jacobus Sylvius, the teacher of Vesalius, believed that Galen's anatomy was infallible and that any progress in knowledge beyond Galen was impossible. Sylvius became one of the fiercest opponents of Vesalius, accusing him of squandering the truths and calling those who dared to follow his rogue student "two-legged asses."

Although there was much opposition surrounding his work, Vesalius's *Fabric* wasn't disregarded by everyone. In fact, it was responsible for influencing a young medical student who would go on to transform the study of medicine forever.

. . .

A typical dissection auditorium of the sixteenth century gives us a picture of the tradition in which anatomy training was imparted to medical students. Professors of anatomy and surgery conducted their classrooms with theatrical elegance. Mirroring the same fervor of an elaborate religious service, incense was burned and fragrant oils were spattered in the halls. Tranquil melodies would fill the auditorium as lute players paraded into the theater, taking their seats around the dissection table. The head porter, the last to enter the room, would demand absolute silence. The distinguished professor, dressed in his finest purple and gold robes, would make his way to a throne of carved wood next to the dissection table, and two assistants would take their seats on carved wooden chairs beside him.

The professor would then address his eager audience:

> The exposition of anatomy is sacred and divine, it must be approached in the same spirit and mind as divine service, since it bears witness to the power, goodness, and wisdom of God. . . . Such marvels of nature should not lie hidden from us, so we shall now reveal them.

. . .

Sixty-five years after Vesalius became the University of Pauda's professor of anatomy and surgery, the school educated William Harvey. Galen's ideas, now sixteen centuries old, continued to form the basis of the medical curriculum. Harvey, like other students, was tasked with memorizing these many theories to become a physician.

"Why doth a woman sometimes conceive twins?" the tutor would demand.

"According to Galen," the sincere student might have answered, "because there is more than one receptacle of seed in the womb."

Upon graduation in 1602, Harvey was appointed as an anatomy lecturer, and he relied upon the hands-on dissection modeled by Vesalius as the precedent for his own teaching style. Yet Harvey was different from his predecessors in that he tried to show not only the structure but also the function and purpose of each part of the body during his lessons.

Harvey performed intricate dissections and then utilized illustrators to delineate various parts of the organs for his classes. He presented learning methods no one dared to follow at the time; he encouraged students to trust their own eyes, even if what they saw defied what they had been taught by generations past. He took a bold stance, proclaiming that ancients were fallible.

Like Vesalius, Harvey continued to debunk some of Galen's most prominent theories. One of these theories was Galen's idea that blood is consumed by the organs it nourishes. Despite this, more than 70 years after Vesalius began to pave the way for new and improved knowledge of anatomy, conservative physicians remained loyal to the teachings of Galen, despite the obvious shortcomings. His theories, while rejected by the masses, introduced a proper understanding of our innards that would go on to change the entire landscape of medicine.

Harvey was lucky to have been educated at a time in history when Galileo Galilei was the most popular teacher at the University of Padua. Galileo was a rebel of his time from early on, being a self-identified "pious Roman Catholic" who fathered three children out of wedlock. Though he was invigorated by a passion for mathematics, his father impelled him instead to study medicine, since physicians at the time earned substantially more money. He caved to his father's persuasion and enrolled for a medical degree. It only took one accidental geometry class, though, for Galileo to drop medicine and choose mathematics as his course of study.

In 1581, when he entered the University of Pisa, Galileo noticed a chandelier in one of the buildings on campus that swung in regular intervals. He likened it to the rhythm of his heartbeat: The chandelier, no matter how far it swung, always took the same amount of time to swing back. He started seeing similarities in human biology and man-made machines. Being fascinated by mathematics, his focus was not on the rhythmic beating of the heart but on the geometry of the swinging pendulum. Had he stuck to his father's dream of studying medicine, Galileo might have changed the landscape of medical knowledge like no other. Nevertheless, by transforming how we understood the world around us, he set a precedent for generations to come not only in astronomy, but across the study of science in general.

At the time of Galileo's study, the Aristotelian theory of the sun circling the Earth was in vogue. The Catholic Church, by adopting some of the ancient Greek doctrines into its theology, insisted that the Earth was the center of the universe and that everything revolved around it. Aristotle left a legacy so influential that for nearly 20 centuries no one dared to question his theories. Galileo was determined to disprove this long-held notion, and, in 1615, he submitted his detailed work supporting the Copernican model (that the sun is the center, not the Earth) to the Roman Inquisition.

A commission called his theory "foolish and absurd" and claimed that it was suspect of heresy. The biggest offense to the church was that Galileo put forth and defended a theory after the Holy Scripture declared the contrary. Guarding the authority of the written word was taken very seriously. For spreading "dangerous new ideas" that would threaten the very foundation of the most popular faith, he was sentenced to a life of house arrest and ordered to read seven penitential psalms once a week for three years. His daughter fought against this punishment and eventually received permission to take it upon herself.

Nevertheless, his work helped further the separation of science from both philosophy and dogma—a necessary step in the progression of human thought. "I wanted people to understand," he agonized, "that nature gave them eyes to see her works, but also brains to make them capable of understanding them." Disgruntled by society's fears to question the status quo, he encouraged his students to reach beyond what was known at the time.

Galileo's influence probably gave young Harvey the necessary courage to boldly publish his observations against dogma that still supported Galen's inaccurate theories. However, there was another obstacle with which Harvey had to contend. At the time, though mathematics and physics were considered studies of science, medicine still fell under the authority of theology.

A prime example of this was the life and discoveries of Michael Servetus. He was the first European to describe pulmonary circulation and to accurately detail the anatomy of several parts of the brain. While these ideas were considered to be accurate and thus challenged the incorrect teachings of Galen, Servetus didn't gain much recognition because he wasn't able to separate his medical and theological writings. Regrettably, his medical findings appeared in his theological text, *The Restoration of Christianity*.

Most copies of the book were burned shortly after its publication in 1553 because of the persecution of Servetus by religious authorities. Despite his contributions to the field of medicine, Servetus's achievements were shadowed by his devout theological beliefs. His firm rejection of the concept of the Holy Trinity is what sparked the vicious conflict. Servetus believed the Trinity wasn't a Biblical idea, having arisen instead from Greek philosophers. He tried to reason with orthodoxy, intending to rid Christianity of the Trinity to make the religion more welcoming to followers of Judaism and Islam, who believed in the idea of one unified God. Tragically, Servetus was burned alive for his beliefs upon a pyre of his own books less than a year after publication.

The orthodoxy didn't even spare the dead. A few years after Servetus was burned, a professor of surgery in Bologna, Italy, named Gasparo Tagliacozzi created a milestone in the field of surgery. In 1557, Tagliacozzi described his innovative surgical methods for correcting abnormalities of the nose, lip, and ear using a technique that involved removing a flap of skin from the upper arm of a patient and attaching it to the open site of the deformity, often the nose. The arm would then be immobilized, anchored to the patient's head with splints, thus restoring circulation and healing. Once the new nose was firmly attached to the face, Tagliacozzi would carefully detach the flap from the arm.

He described his techniques in *De Curtorum Chirurgia per Insitionem*

(*On the Surgery of Mutilation by Grafting*) in 1597 and perfectly summarized the goals of reconstructive surgery:

> We restore, rebuild, and make whole those parts which nature
> hath given, but which fortune has taken away. Not so much that
> it may delight the eye, but that it might buoy up the spirit and
> help the mind of the afflicted.

Tagliacozzi went on to perform other reconstructive operations. One surgery involved the repair of an area of bone loss in the skull of a Russian soldier using a piece of dog skull. Though the operation was successful, Tagliacozzi was condemned by the church for interfering with "God's handiwork." The church ordered removal of the healthy-appearing bone graft *after* it was firmly fused in the head of the Russian. The church was so dismayed by Tagliacozzi's violation of the Canon law that after his death his remains were dug up and reburied in unconsecrated ground.

Reconstructive surgery was eventually banned, and Tagliacozzi's techniques had to lie dormant for three centuries until they were rediscovered by German surgeons in the 1800s.

. . .

People truly believed what a religious authority preached, and so did the authorities doing the preaching. More than simply believing their own dogma, theologians "knew" their beliefs were true in the same way that modern scientists know certain realities to be true. Society was brainwashed under the sweeping influence of early theologians.

Heretics were persecuted not simply out of hatred or malice but as an act of benevolence. Torturing and even burning heretics, for example, was considered a righteous act. It was a means of purging someone of their sins and done only with the best intention of saving them from eternal damnation. Pious authorities did this in the same spirit of a surgeon who's very sorry she has to make a patient undergo an extremely painful amputation of an infected leg. It may be a tough reality, but it will save a life.

To the strictly religious, free-thinking was considered a heresy, an affliction and symptom of a disease. To "cure" him or her of this, the person would first be reasoned with. If this didn't work, then religious authorities would move on to deprive the individual of certain civil rights, impose excommunication, or even commit to corporeal punishment. And if those didn't work, the next step was to hang or burn the offending individual—a last resort that not only served as a warning to others, but also offered a pious hope that the experience would finally enable the heretic to—quite literally—"see the light."

Such was the state of affairs when the scientific spirit was in its nascent stages. And scientific innovation may have remained thwarted if not for a few key individuals who persevered despite the potential for disastrous personal and professional consequences.

. . .

Just as 1543 was a landmark year for the simultaneous publications of works by Copernicus and Vesalius, 1668 was a landmark year for another invention that would forever change the way we understood ourselves—both inside and out. In 1668, Isaac Newton improved on Galileo's refracting telescope by inventing a better version. This new reflecting telescope provided a much closer and clearer view of the cosmos. The gigantic modern telescopes used in cosmological research today are merely enhanced versions of the original Newtonian scope. Months after he perfected his instrument, Italian physician and professor of Medicine at the University of Pisa Marcello Malpighi published a groundbreaking work on blood circulation through his microscopic studies of lungs.

While the telescope revolutionized how we thought about the universe, the microscope transformed what we understood about our inner world. The microscope allowed us to expand upon Harvey's anatomical exposition by directly witnessing how the entire body is honeycombed with minute capillary blood vessels connecting the arteries to the veins beneath our skin. The instrument filled the gaps in knowledge about our inner world like never before.

Accidentally invented by a Dutch optician after he got two lenses stuck in a tube, the microscope was commercialized by Antony van Leeuwenhoek, who's historically tied to the instrument as the first man to see his sperm up close and personal. Having realized that our perceptive capacities are limited, a frenzy of inventions occurred in the seventeenth century to augment our observation, including the spectroscope, the telescope, the gyroscope, and the thermoscope.

Around this time, Western physicians were in a race to discover the next body part. Thomas Willis discovered a loop of blood vessels in the base of the brain and named it the Circle of Willis. The Eustachian tube connecting the middle ear to the pharynx was named after Bartolommeo Eustachio, while Fallopian tubes bear the name of Gabriele Fallopio. Cowper's glands in males and their complementary Bartholin glands in females were named after William Cowper and Casper Bartholin, respectively. We saw Broca's area in the brain, Descemet's membrane in the cornea, the Golgi apparatus in the cell. Whoever uncovered a medical discovery named it after themselves.

The invention of instruments offered confidence that we'd finally discovered all there was to understand about our bodies. In reality, many of the theories to explain illnesses were still only speculative. Instruments to observe even the smallest aspects of our anatomy were insufficient in painting a complete picture. Many bodily functions remained an enigma, hard to read, and, ultimately, unfathomable.

At the time, conservative elements in both the East and West were strongly restricting the mobility of thought by proposing limits to human intellect. According to sixteenth-century preachers, "God hath appointed every man his degree and office, within the limits whereof it behoveth him to keep himself." Society was coerced into believing that anything self-serving was immoral.

Adding to the theological stronghold, another tradition became an unrelenting obligation. For centuries, uncertainties in medicine were resolved simply by senior physicians touting, "in my experience" or "it was said so." Graduating from medical training meant perfecting the theories and philosophies of predecessors. Physicians took pride in this passed-on wisdom—apprentice doctors couldn't wait to earn the credence necessary to establish this level of authority, and doctors emerged as guardians of prevailing doctrines.

Medicine's past is not often a focus in medical schools today, frankly because there is little of which to be proud. We attributed glorified theories to many self-limiting illnesses, taking credit for the body's natural healing abilities. Though there were significant and transformative breakthroughs along the way, the history of medicine is not a testament to seekers of truthful knowledge from across cultures in centuries past. Instead, it's a catalogue of callous hysteria sprinkled with mere glimpses of logic and good-intentioned reason.

To break the iron mold created by centuries of dogma, we had to unscript the entire thought process laid down by our predecessors. The fate of humanity hinged on a breakthrough that would transform how we study nature and ourselves. All that we believed as hard fact for millennia was about to be put to the test.

PART TWO

BRAVE NEW WORLD

"They perforated the chest on one or both sides to learn how the lungs functioned. They strangled the blood supply to organs by tying off arteries to explore how tissues reacted to lack of nutrition. Scientists became more and more creative—and more and more daring— in their attempts to grasp bodily functions using hard facts."

CHAPTER *4*

THE WONDROUS MACHINE

> You feel like an object on a conveyor belt. You don't feel human.
> Medical science has decided, that's the way it is.
>
> —A PATIENT'S EXPERIENCE DURING HOSPITALIZATION

One afternoon during Walter Stephenson's lengthy recovery, just before wrapping up my rounds, I asked, as I always did, if he had any questions. He nodded, gathering his thoughts, as I stepped to the end of his bed to face him.

He looked in my direction and asked, "Why do you all see me as just . . . as a collection of diseases?"

I encouraged him to explain what he meant, and he shared that at times it felt more like his physicians were there to treat his disease as its own entity, not as if it existed in a person with priorities, beliefs, and emotions that also deserved consideration.

I paused to think about this. Walter was right. Each specialist on his care team, myself included, had a plan to tackle Walter's disease through our own area of expertise. We saw Walter—as we see many of our patients—as an intricate machine with faulty parts that needed to be fixed. This doesn't mean that we didn't see Walter as a human with human needs, but when it specifically came to our medical approach, we were each solving our own puzzles.

If a health issue is simple, most people accept and perhaps even welcome this mindset—this is the way that many medical professionals have been trained to do our jobs. But when afflicted with multiple medical problems, such as the case with Walter, this can be harder to reconcile. During his extended hospital stay, Walter was bounced between specialists, hearing varying opinions about how to treat the parts of his internal machinery that weren't working properly. At times, he felt like his voice went unheard, or when it was, that treatment wasn't consistent among specialists. It's no surprise, then, that he sometimes felt dejected or even dehumanized.

As a medical student, I was trained to see the human body as a wondrous machine. A complex instrument comprised of smaller interconnected machines, like a factory. But unlike man-made technology, the parts comprising the human body are less rigid. The components that make up the engine of a car or the hardware of a computer work together in a way that's inflexible. If too much variance is introduced, if pieces are swapped out or missing, the machine breaks. The same can't be said, however, of the human body. Despite innumerable fluctuations—some of which are unforeseen—the body is able to keep itself stable through a system of feedback controls that regulate its internal environment and achieve homeostasis. It's only when abnormalities become too great that we experience failures in the operation of our bodies in the form of disease.

From a simplistic view, our bodies are nothing but a fantastic tube with a ganglion at one end that acts as a sensory unit and an outlet at the other end to eliminate processed waste. Everything in between is a complicated, ever-evolving conglomerate of cannulas and pulleys connected by circuitry and propelled by highly specialized chemicals flowing through tortuous conduits—a wondrous machine. In fact, I don't know any other way of tackling the human body when it comes to detecting and treating a physical illness, but I can also see how this might create apprehension from the other side of the bed from a patient's point of view.

And here's why: Even as a doctor, when I see myself in the mirror, I don't see my body as a glorious machine. I see it as an intelligence in an elaborate ecosystem that works in communion with innumerable other ecosystems, big and small, beyond its boundaries. I see myself as a fertile ground full of emotions, beliefs, preferences, choices, insights, memories, potentials, and so much more.

But when it comes to approaching health and sickness, this can't always be my approach. If there's a blockage in a vessel in a person's heart, we clean it up and put in a stent or perform a bypass, taking a piece of similar blood vessel from elsewhere and patching up the problem area. Broken bones become mended again after being supported by screws and plates. Doctors function as mechanics—when something is wrong, we find it and fix it.

Physicians and biologists use the term "mechanism" liberally in describing a disease process or an organic function. We describe our bodies as being made up of "parts" instead of referring to them as "features." The terminology has become so ubiquitous that modern-day physicians don't even realize that their understanding of the human body as a complicated machine is a relatively new idea.

CHAPTER 5

PARADIGM SHIFT

I'm not interested in preserving the status quo. I want to overthrow it.
—NICCOLÒ MACHIAVELLI, ITALIAN RENAISSANCE PHILOSOPHER

In a radical departure from tradition, a few natural philosophers in seventeenth-century Western Europe grew discontented with the Greek view of the world. Chemists tried and failed to find any evidence of a special "life force" that distinguished living entities from inorganic matter. Some philosophers even started to distance themselves from the idea of an all-powerful, sovereign creator involved in day-to-day activities. This shift, which became overwhelmingly important for the further development of human thought, was initiated and propagated by two towering figures of the time: Francis Bacon and René Descartes.

Francis Bacon (1561–1626) touched medicine at several points, predominantly regarding the introduction of methods to study human physiology. It was primarily because of Bacon that the seventeenth century became the bedrock of experimental studies. Bacon started a revolution in understanding the natural world by changing the face of exploration through his fearless approach. He became convinced that the only types of theories worth considering were ones that could be put to the test.

The crux of his idea lay in the basic logic that the accumulation of facts by way of mere observation, which had been the method used for centuries prior, was not sufficient to study nature. In modern times, we take this understanding entirely for granted, but this was a radical notion then. This new method of investigation employed reasoning from a part to a whole, from the elemental to the general, and this approach became the guiding spirit of all scientific studies for centuries to follow.

Although this idea may be touched upon in ancient and medieval periods, Bacon was the first to formalize a method for investigating nature. His idea was deceptively simple yet inherently so profound that no force could withstand its logic. He proclaimed that: "My way of discovering knowledge performs everything by the surest rules." He cast aside former thinkers like Plato, rejecting the practice of combining facts of nature with the untestable, subjective doctrines of theology and Greek philosophy. In his famous text on education, *The Advancement of Learning* (1605), Bacon argued that medicine had progressed little, if at all, during this time, as it relied too heavily on antiquated authorities. He was dedicated to objectivity and an unbiased examination of nature, claiming that: "All depends on keeping the eye steadily fixed on the facts of nature, and so receiving their images simply as they are."

He believed that knowledge is not an opinion, but a work that must be verified. "Old methods should die," wrote Francis Bacon, proposing methods for a new beginning. Here, for the first time, was the voice and tone of modern science. Francis Bacon actually called this the "new philosophy." This was different from anything that came before it because it prioritized practice rather than theory. This approach focused on search of proof instead of a doctrine, putting emphasis on something concrete and provable as opposed to speculation.

Bacon suggested that even the human body could be subjected to experimentation. Although he proudly proposed the new method of study, there was another task that remained unfulfilled. He had to overthrow the immutable philosophical concepts that his predecessors firmly established. Without this step, his scientific method would be quickly rejected.

Much of the philosophical basis of medical practice dates back to the writings of Aristotle and, to a lesser degree, Plato. Aristotle's philosophy that men didn't know a thing until they had grasped the *why* of it (the first cause, or the Prime Mover) was still very much a part of students' curriculum.

This was, in fact, the running theme across all medical training in the West well into the seventeenth century. One student described the instructors of the University of Padua as "philosophers into whom Aristotle seemed to have migrated."

Physicians, as students of philosophy, were also schooled in the idea of the soul being the immutable force that determines all vital functions of the body. Medical education was imparted in religious institutions, and philosophy was a required course for medical students. Aristotle's Prime Mover, interpreted as the soul or spirit by successive philosophers and theologians, hindered experiments on the human body. The future of experimental biology hinged on eliminating the concept of the soul from the mind of every biologist, medical student, and practicing physician.

Bacon tried to disavow this concept of the soul using Galileo's theory that natural philosophy ought to be based on "sensory experience and necessary demonstration" rather than an abstract exploration of the *why* of things. Bacon reasoned that the essence of something is always beyond our comprehension, and seeking the first cause is akin to pursing a "phantom" (meaning the soul). Scientists should be concerned with the immediate causes of a disease, he emphasized.

For the scientific method to advance without being dragged back into the Dark Ages, he had to, once and for all, settle the theory of the soul being the supreme commander of all vital actions. Bacon needed additional support in undertaking this mammoth task of transforming the natural philosopher into a man of science. The link between these two roles was so deeply rooted into our understanding that even to this day the title PhD—Doctor of Philosophy—is given to scientists after years of pursuing scientific research in academia. The degree isn't termed a "Doctor of Science," because for centuries doctoral candidates were required to study philosophy before they could advance to a more specialized area of focus. We've carried forward this title even though mastering philosophy is no longer a requisite part of the curriculum.

As science shifted to the forefront, Bacon found the well-needed support in another soaring giant who singularly changed our idea of ourselves and that of the natural world by stubbornly promoting absolute freedom of the authority of previous philosophers.

. . .

The French philosopher René Descartes (1596–1650) was fascinated by mechanical clocks. He pondered:

> Could the universe have been devised by a sort of industrious watch-maker deity? Could it be similar to a clock rather than the divine animated being imagined by natural philosophers down the centuries? That is, might not the world be bereft of spirits and invisible forces and run mechanically or automatically like the actions and motions of a clock?

His philosophical theories were shaped by an insight that once woke him up in the middle of the night—the key to the universe is its mathematical order. Descartes wondered, "might our bodies be merely machine-like, no different than the man-made ones?" After much contemplation, he concluded, "My thought . . . compares a sick man and an ill-made clock with my idea of a healthy man and a well-made clock."

Although this idea is primarily attributed to Descartes, this is not an entirely new concept. In fact, we can see this mechanistic analogy dating back to the fifteenth century in the works of Leonardo da Vinci. He was a polymath like some of his contemporaries, self-trained in engineering, mathematics, medicine, anatomy, painting, and astronomy. While meticulously recording the shape and function of various tissues during his elaborate human dissections, he also became fascinated with the flight of birds and dreamed of building a human-powered flying machine. Describing the mechanics of flying at one point in his *Codex on the Flight of Birds*, he wrote, "The *engine* of these wings, that is the bird's body, overcomes the resistance of the air and advances. . . . " He formulated elaborate descriptions on the flight of birds using the principles of "Elements of Machinery" and drew prototypes of how this might be applied to humans.

But da Vinci was too ahead of his time. Born out of wedlock, which was highly taboo in his era, he was not taken seriously. His ideas were cast away as the mindless preoccupations of a poor, wandering artist. Although there are no records to prove this, it's possible that da Vinci's ideas influenced the young Descartes.

As one of the first philosophers to defend Harvey's circulation theory in print, Descartes drew many metaphors from the mechanical world to explain the various bodily functions. In his *Discourse on Method* in 1637, Descartes described the heart as a mechanical pump, comparing it to a combustion engine driven by a series of explosions occurring in regular intervals, as though by clockwork. The entire current-day practice of medicine is based on this idea. The heart, for instance, is treated as a mechanical pump, a vital part of the corporeal machinery, where cardiologists are its plumbers and electro-physiologists are its electricians.

This approach—that of comparing the body to a machine—made

it much easier to study its parts. In his *Discourse on Method*, René Descartes instructs: "Divide each difficulty into as many parts as is feasible and necessary to resolve it," urging readers to construct their thoughts in such an order that, by commencing with objects from the simplest and easiest to know, they will ascend little by little, step by step, to the knowledge of the more complex.

The knottier problem that Descartes belabored most of his life was the interpretation of the relationship between soul and matter. Although Descartes didn't entirely reject the populist perception of the soul as the foundation of material life, he entertained a rational version. He frequently equated the soul to the mind where all our thoughts are formed. He gave an exact anatomical location of the soul in a tiny organ in the center of our brain, somewhere midway between our ears and behind the center of our eyes, called the Pineal gland, which he believed to be the "seat of the soul." By offering a more tangible location of the soul, Descartes felt that he provided an objective reality to the abstract idea.

In Descartes's time, it was not unusual to associate a metaphysical ideal or an abstract feeling with an organ. For instance, valor and honesty were associated with heart, heat with the stomach, irritability with the liver, and melancholy with the spleen. But to assign the soul itself to a specific organ was unconventional even to those who rallied behind Descartes's ideas. Nevertheless, his insistence on the absolute freedom of thought ushered in a new age of emancipation from dogma.

· · ·

As Bacon denounced the first-cause principle of Aristotle using his scientific method, Descartes diminished the position of the soul as the Prime Mover of all human actions using his logic. While one laid the foundation of the scientific inquiry, the other gave the necessary impetus, without which the scientific method could never have seen fruition.

Their writings ushered in a new world of thought, breaking Aristotle's[1] and Galen's long holds.

It all came down to closing a critical loophole in Aristotle's formalized system of reasoning established in the fourth century. In his theories, Aristotle failed to create a language that enabled him (or his followers) to objectively describe the knowable aspects of the world, as well as to test theories by experimentation. As a result, the long-standing influence of some of the Aristotelian doctrines began to crumble.

The period between the seventeenth and eighteenth centuries was considered the Age of Enlightenment, though not in the spiritual sense; the opposite, in fact, was true, and the time was typified by questioning authority. Immanuel Kant, who is considered the central figure of modern philosophy, declared, "Dare to be wise" as the motto of this era. A lack of courage to challenge those in power was viewed as a weakness, and in the quest to advance human knowledge, emerging from our self-incurred immaturity was considered a triumph of reason over dogma.

The dawn of the eighteenth century brought with it the idea of a mechanical universe governed by the laws of physics, as opposed to a universe created by an all-powerful spiritual being. Explaining natural phenomena through theories that hinged on prophecies and revelations became an increasingly discredited practice among many scholarly communities. This era was marked by the rise of individual free-thinkers who would change our understanding of our universe with such fierce conviction that when they showed proof of their ideas, no religious or philosophical authorities could stand in their way.

Even artists were influenced by the mechanical disposition of the universe. Alexander Pope, an influential eighteenth-century English

---

1   Despite his achievements in many areas of philosophy, Aristotle's theories were considered by many
      to have held back scientific advancement considerably. Bertrand Russell observed that "almost
      every serious intellectual advance has had to begin with an attack on some Aristotelian doctrine."
      (Bertrand Russell, *A History of Western Philosophy*, Simon & Schuster, 1972)

poet, spent his life introspecting mankind's place in the universe and its relationship with God. Like many of his contemporaries who were influenced by Descartes, Pope believed in the existence of a God who had created and presided over a physical universe that functioned like a vast clockwork mechanism. The idea of God wasn't cast aside, but the role was reassigned to one more similar to a watchmaker.

When the iron-fisted grip of Aristotelian theories on natural philosophy eventually gave way to scientific reason, the undisputed doctrines were finally put to rest. For instance, prominent seventeenth-century English philosopher Thomas Hobbes spread his understanding of humans as *matter in motion*, meaning we obey the same physical laws of mechanics as other objects.

Eventually, the influential thinkers would drop the idea of God altogether in their studies, keeping to the laws of nature to advance their exploration. Concepts such as the soul or spirit were outside the purview of science, they declared, because the hypothesis of God was not verifiable.

With progressive materialization of the body, structures and functions were explained in terms of "mechanisms." This approach contributed to the tendency to treat specific illnesses localized to particular organs, the dawn of a disease-centered approach to medicine. For clinicians, this move essentially meant casting aside 2,000 years of wisdom for a new methodology.

Such a radical overhaul meant future doctors would not even know what a "humor" was, and that Galen's legacy in medicine would all but disappear. Pythagoras, the forefather of humoral theory would not be remembered for his contributions to medicine. Medical students of the future would not know that Hippocrates, famous for his oath and introducing rational thinking into medicine, actually practiced medicine based on the humoral theory, relying heavily on the healing power of nature. Almost all of the accepted wisdom of medicine would fade quietly into a forgotten past.

For the physician to accept this radical view, there was one major hurdle. While material scientists had conceived a method to test their theories using a mechanistic approach, the medical community was left clueless as to how to experimentally study life forms the same way.

Scientists studying inorganic phenomena—like a chemist exploring the composition of matter—could control an experiment to test their hypothesis. A biologist, on the other hand, couldn't control the innumerable variables that interfere with the natural condition of vital processes in the human body.

As a result, physicians were left in limbo when trying to discover how and why illness strikes. A whole new approach to medicine was around the corner. A decision needed to be reached by the medical community. This shift had tremendous implications that would transform the very substance of medicine. This was the biggest decision the medical community had yet to face, and the consequences of this conceptual leap would be judged by generations to come.

CHAPTER 6

EMERGENCE OF A NEW SENTIMENT

> Life is a similar process in cabbages and kings; I choose to work
> on cabbages because they are cheaper and easier to come by.
>
> —ALBERT SZENT-GYÖRGYI, 1937 NOBEL PRIZE IN PHYSIOLOGY
> RECIPIENT, ON WHY HE DOESN'T EXPERIMENT ON HUMANS

In 1645, an informal group of natural philosophers were inspired by the "new science" and began holding secret, late-evening meetings. They called themselves "The Invisible College." The group included one particularly young chemist, Robert Boyle. Boyle went on to author 42 books, 30 of which were scientific treatises. In *The Sceptical Chymist* (1661), Boyle attacked the Aristotelian theory of the four elements (earth, air, fire, and water). According to Boyle, natural phenomena were explained not by Aristotelian elements, but by the motion and organization of primary gas particles in the air.

Although he was a religious man, his views of faith were transformed by the rationalist movement of the century. Influenced by Descartes, Boyle believed nature to be a clock-like mechanism that works according to certain physical laws set in motion by a creator.

In his experiments, Boyle noted that when placed in a chamber, birds and mice die promptly when air is removed. He remarked that "We may suppose that there is in the air a little vital Quintessence . . . which serves to the refreshment and restoration of our vital spirits." He didn't stop there, but went on to add that his idea "should not be barely asserted but explicated and proved."

Fifteen years after its inception, The Invisible College and similar groups coalesced into a single structured organization designed to promote the era's scientific spirit. This group came to be called "The Royal Society," which was officially founded in 1660. The Royal Society repeatedly said that it was the impetus of Francis Bacon's writings that led to its formation. It became one of the world's most influential scientific societies.

· · ·

In exploring how the world works, thinkers were divided into two camps. The idealists believed that there was a creative force behind the universe, and that everything works according to a grand plan. To them, the universe was seen as a cosmic theater, "God's sensorium." On a quest to understand the creator's mind, they believed that by discovering the laws of nature, we would one day discover its inner workings. Nicolaus Copernicus, Galileo Galilei, Leonardo da Vinci, Robert Boyle, Isaac Newton, Carl Linnaeus, William Harvey, and Gregor Mendel were counted among this group. Many of these individuals would comb the scriptures for clues, meditate upon the theories of ancient philosophers, and immerse themselves in obscure alchemical experiments. In spite of this, they would also probe the latest scientific publications with utmost rigor. Robert Boyle believed that there were no conflicts between science and the Bible, but if one was found, it was either due to an error in our experiment or an incorrect interpretation of Scripture. This was a time when God was a part of "science."

The skeptics, on the other hand, held that there might have been a grand creator organizing the workings of nature, but we would never know that because we could not prove the existence of such a force. Our human pursuit was not to seek out that potential truth, but to use our intellect to penetrate the inner workings of nature. Unlike the theists who had a grand creator to explain every working of nature, the skeptics didn't see a creator's existence as a matter of necessity to explain everything. The belief that a supreme commander was holding all the threads of a person's fate was simply too autocratic.

Skeptics detested the idea of a powerful divine being watching and judging every aspect of human activity, all the way down to our innermost feelings and thoughts. The question "*How did consciousness arise from brute matter?*" continued to puzzle them. Despite this, they resisted the temptation of allowing metaphysical beliefs to fog their intellect. To them, knowledge is derived from our sensory experience of the world. They were more inclined to pursue how individual things and forces in nature interacted. When it came to the ultimate explanation of existential questions, such as *why* the world existed or *why* there was suffering, a genuine skeptic maintained restraint. Seeking meaning in things was not their quest, and these beliefs became the foundation of scientific inquiry.

In 1802, Napoleon Bonaparte was presented the *Traité de mécanique céleste*—a five-volume work that detailed the workings of the solar system—by its author, French mathematician Laplace. Napoleon taunted him that he had neglected to mention God in the books, stating, "Monsieur Laplace, they tell me you have written this large book on the system of the universe, and have never even mentioned its Creator." Laplace had a famous retort: "Sire, I have no need of that hypothesis."

To an empiricist,[1] it doesn't matter if a statement *sounded* meaningful; statements like "God moves all things" or "spirit controls matter" fell empty without proof. They needed to be verified. This thinking was the point of departure from the age-old tradition of conformity to dogma.

Over time, the word *scientific* became synonymous with *skeptic*. The Age of Enlightenment saw the rise of this latter group, the free-thinkers.

. . .

Seventeenth-century physicians mustered courage and boldly questioned why medicine was lagging behind the sciences of inert matter. By then, physicists and chemists learned an enormous amount (compared to their medieval counterparts) about how the world worked in an extremely short period of time.

Astronomy was progressing in an era when physiology remained relatively unknown. Many conceivable aspects of nature were being reduced to verifiable mechanisms. And an array of other mechanisms were explained by their relationships to one another, providing a glimpse into how the universe operated. Galileo reduced the Earth, once center of the universe, to the rank of a humble satellite of the sun. Newton recognized that the same force responsible for an apple falling also kept the moon in orbit. Robert Boyle separated alchemy from chemistry and established its status as science. Blaise Pascal invented the first mechanical calculator that was used in Europe and then around the world. William Gilbert laid the foundations of the theories of electricity and magnetism.

Physicists and chemists were advancing their understanding of nature by creating optimal conditions in which certain phenomena

---

1   Empiricism is the theory that asserts the role of evidence in all matters of inquiry. Every proposition must be put to test. I find it ironic that these empiricists decidedly chose not to test the truth in the statement that *knowledge comes only or primarily from sensory experience*. This, in a sense, became accepted wisdom of empiricists.

could be experimentally tested. Biologists became convinced they could do the same. Life viewed as a "chemical accident" was catching up across all disciplines of science. To unravel the mysteries of human biology, physiologists allied themselves with chemists and physicists.

Well aware that biology is complex and cannot be studied en bloc, the founders of the scientific method began their analysis of bodily mechanisms by separating them experimentally into distinct and simple parts. The rationale was that to observe any biological phenomenon, it first must be reduced to a state of simplicity that we could grasp. Scientific circles came to the conclusion that the field of medicine could only advance using the same methodical experimentation employed by inorganic sciences.

In utilizing this approach, Giovanni Borelli of Italy proved that the laws of inorganic sciences offered the key to the body's operations. Initially trained in mathematics and physics, the seventeenth-century polymath undertook studies in medicine. He applied principles of material sciences to understand human physiology. He was able to meticulously study individual functions such as muscle behavior, gland secretions, respiration, movements of the heart, and neural responses. Borelli's main contribution was his remarkable observations of birds in flight, fish swimming, muscular contraction, the mechanics of breathing, and a host of similar subjects in which he attempted to define the functions of the human body. In Borelli's highly innovative work, physics and chemistry jointly promised to unravel the secrets of life.

This idea laid the foundation of future research in medicine. "The laws of chemistry and physics are identical in the world of living things and in that of inanimate matter," declared nineteenth-century physiologist Claude Bernard.

A classic archetype of how physicists and biologists came together to unravel the mysteries of human organism is the story of the double helix, the molecule of DNA. Francis Crick was a physicist and James Watson was a molecular biologist. On a winter morning in February of 1953, Crick announced the discovery by walking into their nearby Eagle Pub and blurting out, "We have found the secret of life." Without the aid of the physicist, the biologist could not have discovered DNA, which was the most important medical discovery at the time.

. . .

As the eighteenth-century medical profession was increasingly emancipated from the stronghold of theology, a renewed worldview was born. Humankind was indisputably justified in testing animals and every other living thing. The guilt of using subordinate life forms for human experiments was lifted off the shoulders of biologists who were eager to explore.

With all living entities able to become instruments in scientific study, biologists could breathe freely from centuries-old oppressive dogma for the first time. By liberally experimenting on animals and humans, biologists were able to discover inner workings of the body that had remained obscured for hundreds of years. Eager scientists rushed to sever the spinal cord at different levels, enabling the systematic study of various nerve actions. They perforated the chest on one or both sides to learn how the lungs functioned. They strangled the blood supply to organs by tying off arteries to explore how tissues reacted to lack of nutrition. Scientists became more and more creative—and more and more daring—in their attempts to grasp bodily functions using hard facts.

Biologists found this method of investigating nature extremely rewarding. Since their approach was harder to systematize in medicine than in other scientific fields, an order was established among the different processes of investigation. Increasing the power of perception by using tools or techniques to penetrate the body, isolate regions of study, and examine the otherwise hidden territories became a requirement.

Experimentation permitted investigators to intervene, even if that meant altering or even destroying their given area of study in an effort to fully understand the part it played in the whole.

Creating conditions suitable for testing became the most vital step in utilizing the scientific method. Scientists called this *controlled* experimentation. The idea behind this arrangement is simple: The results of a test should, in theory, always present in the same way if the conditions are similar. If results between two scientists differed, these differences were explained by inconsistencies in the experimental conditions. This approach was widely advocated through examples: If a sciatic nerve is cut, and all conditions are constant, then the subject's leg will become paralyzed. This study could be reproduced over and over again and would yield the same result.

With the application of experimental methods, medical scientists were uncovering the mysteries of human biology at lightning speed. One of the first to get in the game was Italian anatomist Giovanni Morgagni. He was credited with founding the discipline of pathological anatomy. Morgagni demonstrated that specific diseases were located in specific organs, which was a relatively innovative idea for his time. Marie-François Bichat, a French physiologist, later discovered that diseases attacked tissues rather than whole organs, another game-changer in medical science. His work was so transformative that historian John Lesch wrote: "He has fulfilled the long-standing eighteenth-century ambition to do for physiology and medicine what Newton had done for physics," drawing inspiration from the men of material sciences.

Many advances occurred in diagnostics, too. The Dutch professor Herman Boerhaave began to use the thermometer to record changes in patients' body temperatures in clinical practice. Austrian physician Leopold Auenbrugger spread the importance of tapping on the chest to detect fluid in the lungs. Frenchman René Laënnec made it possible for doctors to listen to internal organs when he invented the stethoscope.

This remained the most important medical invention until Wilhelm Roentgen discovered X-rays in 1895.

Therapeutics experienced a similar path in the 1800s. The English physician Thomas Sydenham proved the use of Peruvian bark for the treatment of malaria. English naval surgeon James Lind demonstrated that citrus fruits cured scurvy. French chemist Pierre Joseph Pelletier isolated colchicine as a treatment for gout. William Withering, a botanist and physician from England, discovered the effectiveness of the foxglove plant in treating heart disorders, which is still used in current-day medical therapeutics. And a British country doctor, Edward Jenner, developed the smallpox vaccine and was credited with having "saved more lives than the work of any other human."

As the founding fathers of North America laid the groundwork of the New World, they made a point to stand behind the scientific method as the only reliable means to examine nature. Thomas Jefferson, the third president of the United States and author of the Declaration of Independence, wrote:

> Bacon, Locke, and Newton. I consider them as the three greatest men that have ever lived, without any exception, and as having laid the foundation of those superstructures which have been raised in the Physical and Moral sciences.

Despite such promising developments, the most popular healing practices were still based on the humoral theories of Hippocrates and Galen. Many new ideologies sprang up, casting the experimental approach as nothing more than a soulless preoccupation.

The West encountered another major hurdle with the rise of the physician-philosopher, a concept that reared its head again during the eighteenth and early nineteenth centuries. Physicians with strong philosophical inclinations started to blend theories of science with the abstractions of metaphysics.

Even after the scientific methodology of Francis Bacon and the mechanistic approach of René Descartes transformed the critical thinking of academic circles, public acceptance was slower to catch on. People demanded simple, easy-to-grasp explanations for diseases in which a healer could instantly do something to cure the ailment. It didn't matter how insubstantial those theories may be.

People were overwhelmed by the astonishing surge in scientific inventions, and many were dissatisfied with the use of "poisons" in medicine. For instance, some expressed displeasure about the treatments of illnesses that used things like mechanically extracted chemicals from plants. Feeling as though this mechanical approach was too extreme, coupled with a widespread impatience from the paucity of new discoveries in medicine, people became drawn to metaphysics. Numerous healing traditions began to spring up locally and snowballed across Europe.

The stream of discoveries fueled by physicists and chemists generated as many new routes of healing in the medical community as it did in metaphysical circuits. Everything from galvanism to the Watt steam engine to the discovery of electricity aided in this effort.

As a result of this new phenomenon, healers with philosophical appetite were synthesizing mechanical concepts discovered by physicists with their own metaphysical theories to explain health and disease. Mystics claimed their knowledge to be superior to the facts obtained from methodical experimentation. People were drawn to these contrived theories, which appealed to emotions rather than to the rational mind. The mystics convinced the public that their understanding of nature was attained directly from supernatural beings, and their many followers in the West agreed with every word. The metaphysical fog had descended on us again.

Sir Kenelm Digby (1601–1665) was known as the "ornament of England" and became one of the most versatile historical figures of the time. He combined the trinity of medicine, philosophy, and religion into a succinct line of thought, with each string of ideas supporting the other. He was popular among metaphysicians who used scientific proof to illustrate religious doctrines, a preoccupation that has continued into contemporary times.

Digby's ascent to fame was the advocacy of his "Powder of Sympathy" through his writings in *A Late Discourse*. Digby recounts that while he was a boy in Florence, a traveling Christian monk gave him a secret powder that could heal wounds at a distance. Years later, his friend James Howel was severely wounded while trying to break up a fight. The wound wouldn't heal for a long time, so Digby was consulted to exercise his "magic" cure. Digby requested the bandages that had first been used to bind Howel's wound. He then dissolved his special powder in water and dipped the dressing into it. Immediately, Howel reported he felt "no more pain" and "a pleasing kind of freshness" in his wounded hand. Digby withdrew the wound dressing from his solution and strangely the pain returned. The dressing was immersed into the solution and allowed to remain there; in a few days, the wound healed. His tales about this so-called enchanted powder became so popular that after his book's first publication in French, it was translated into English, German, and Latin. Digby died on his birthday, and his epitaph reads:

Under this tomb the matchless Digby lies,
Digby the great, the valiant, and the wise:
This age's wonder for his noble parts,
Skilled in six tongues, and learned in all the arts.

The doctrine of *transplantatio morborum* was another philosophy similar to the theory of powder, which was widespread in the seventeenth century. According to this doctrine, ailments and remedies could be transferred from one body to another by the psychosomatic powers of healers. These concepts were loaded with superstition and speculation, yet they constantly challenged the scientific community.

Another popular philosopher-physician was American psychologist John Bovee Dods. Dods came up with his own theory of electricity to explain bodily functions and derangements. He declared:

> Twenty years ago, I discovered electricity to be the connecting link between mind and inert matter. Ever since 1830, I have contended that electricity is . . . the grand agent employed by the Creator to move and govern the universe.

Dods speculated about the most puzzling question of the time. If the mind continually throws off electricity from the brain by its mental operations, then how is the supply kept up—through what source is it introduced into the body? He deferred to physiologists about the mechanical pump function of the heart and framed his own theory of blood circulation to support this metaphysical concept.

He hypothesized that blood in the lungs is electrified with every breath we take and assumes a cherry-red appearance. This "energizing process" purifies the blood and prepares it for circulation. It is then circulated through the nerves and conducted to the brain for use by the mind. He argued that the heart is only a conduit for this process, much like a water tank. The heart does not circulate the blood at all, Dods concluded, which defied the prevailing theories of circulation proved by William Harvey.

Dods was undeniably convincing;[2] he captivated his followers, who in turn believed every detail of his theories. Dods' popularity soared due to his unique way of attracting crowds. He was able to influence several

---

2   Dods' lectures were extremely popular, with high attendance rates, and once published in books, they sold out so quickly that a number of later editions continued to be issued in the next few years. In these lectures, Dods expressed his belief in the power of the agent discovered by Mesmer. He referred to mesmerisms as a "power of God," and attributed the healing work of Jesus with that power. In his lectures, he details six degrees of mesmerism, which included clairvoyance, and discussed surgical uses for them.

politicians and gained much attention through the press. Members of Congress were impressed by his "Electrical Psychology" and felt they needed to better understand what they called "the philosophy of disease." They credited Dods as the discoverer of a new science.

The fundamental reason why many speculations in medicine continued to remain fashionable was mainly because the experimental methods hadn't yet become the universal driver of understanding physiology for the masses.

This whimsical period in medicine enchanted the West until 1865, the year Claude Bernard published his game-changing book *An Introduction to the Study of Experimental Medicine*. This work tried to bring down metaphysical theories of health and disease. We came to the recognition that many common diseases were actually self-limited, i.e., they got better by themselves over time with supportive treatments such as attention to hygiene, proper nursing, regulation of diet, and avoidance of harsh medications. This largely removed the role of superstition and metaphysics from mainstream healing practices. The scientific medical community began to embrace the conviction that, for centuries prior, the greater part of practiced medicine had been largely nonsense.

. . .

In June of 1860, biologist Thomas Huxley (known as "Darwin's Bulldog") and Bishop Samuel Wilberforce debated Darwin's *Origin of Species* at the British Association for Advancement of Science annual meeting, seven months after its publication.

Bishop Wilberforce, dubbed the greatest public speaker of the time, mockingly asked Huxley, "Was it through your grandfather or grandmother that you claimed your descent from a monkey?" Huxley is said to have humbly replied that he would not be ashamed to have a monkey for his ancestor, though he *would* be ashamed to be connected with a man who used his "great gifts" to obscure the truth.

Such humility from scientific proponents inspired those who were already starting to doubt the interests of orthodoxy. Slowly, some of the long-held philosophical and spiritual doctrines were being looked down upon as a form of delusion. New laws upon which the living world operated, in particular Darwin's theory of evolution, rendered the study of life sciences far less mystical. For instance, until the early 1800s, the generally agreed-upon age of the Earth was 10,000 years. By the time Darwin died in 1882, the estimated age of Earth was a whopping 100 million years among scientific circles. Denouncing the all-powerful status of humans once proclaimed by ancients, a profound change occurred in the understanding of who we are and what our place was in the universe. Man was reduced from the unique status as the beloved child of God to a clever monkey. This tug of war between the two world views reached its peak in the nineteenth century.

Even during such unsettled times, a few rare individuals emerged who were both spiritually inclined and scientifically inspired. These individuals didn't find their personal faith to be a serious impediment to their scientific studies, and this sentiment has survived the test of time.

One of these individuals was Cyrill Franz Napp, the abbot (or head monk) of the monastery of St. Thomas in Bruun. Napp worked to turn the monastery into a leading intellectual center where priests included botanists, astronomers, and composers. He sought out bright young men with fervor for learning and strong intellectual abilities to join the monastery. Johann Mendel, who had a flair for discovery, was introduced to Napp by a physics professor from the local university. After entering the priesthood in 1853, Johann's name was changed to Gregor.

Mendel was more than merely an ordinary monk who got lucky. He was a well-trained scientist who studied physics, statistics, chemistry, and physiology at the University of Vienna. He was drawn toward the study of experimental biology but, being financially bereft, joined the priesthood to obtain a free education.

Working like a theoretical physicist, Mendel used mathematical and statistical models to show that there was something within a plant determining its physical properties. Instead of looking up toward the skies for the answers, he conducted methodical experiments to learn more about that "something." It turned out to be the key component of all life—the gene. Decades later, this discovery evolved into an entire science in and of itself: genetics. But Mendel spent just 12 years of his life in scientific study. After Napp's death, he was elected the new abbot of the monastery and gave up his studies in experimental biology. At the age of 45, Mendel accepted full-time duties as the monastic head, a position he retained until his death.

The rediscovery of Mendel's laws of inheritance meant that doctors now had to learn the new science of genes and incorporate this knowledge into their practices. More and more evidence was trickling in to clinics and hospitals that put doctors on the side of reason against superstition, proof against dogma, credibility against quackery, and ultimately sense against nonsense.

The newfound vision of the scientific method was unlike anything seen before in the history of human civilization. It was not comparable to forms of government, religion, education, marriage, or financial institutions, all of which relied on a central authority to function. Without this central authority, social order crumbled. But the scientific method, being an intangible and self-correcting force, was able to inspire enthusiasts who wanted to understand how things worked in nature. Unlike the scriptures, wherein what was mentioned in it was the authority, the scientific method *itself* was what was sovereign. The accumulated knowledge changed over time (also unlike scriptures) as new results were furnished. It self-governed by way of strict criteria and relied only on facts proven through experimentation. The objective of an experimenter was not to preserve his or her theory by seeking only evidence that would support it and setting aside those that may weaken it. The scientific method established new criteria to judge the usefulness of information. It was understood that the wisdom of our ancients must be preserved only as long as it was consistent with observed facts. From this point forward, this impersonal authority went on to dominate human advancement.

The scientific method emerged as the universal equalizer for all those who yearned to study nature. Everyone in the scientific community abides by these dictums, including physicians. In the study of biological phenomena, the scientific method allowed for the reinterpretation of original ideas as unexpected information and facts become available, which may lead to changes in an original theory. In the end, the knowledge of a physician is always subject to change, no matter who discovered what.

PART THREE

BALANCING SCIENCE AND ART

"For the first time in the practice of medicine, a statistical study was used to discredit a medical practice that needed to be subdued because of extravagant claims its creator was making without any factual basis. That creator was ... "

CHAPTER 7

STUDIES, STUDIES, AND MORE STUDIES

To not look at the data is foolish, but to look at the data
as having all the answers is even more foolish.

—TIM KURKJIAN

After finishing medical school in 2001, I enrolled in the MBA program at the University of Missouri. My goal was to gain management skills in the rapidly changing medical marketplace, keeping the door open to potentially become a physician leader later on in my career.

In one class, our Finance professor enthusiastically passed around a *New York Times* article titled "Hormone Replacement Study a Shock to the Medical System." Our assignment was to assess how that hot-button news might affect the bottom-line and reputation of Wyeth, the maker of the popular estrogen replacement drug. "The announcement yesterday," read the July 10, 2002 article, "that a hormone replacement regimen taken by six million American women did more harm than good was met with puzzlement and disbelief by women and their doctors across the country."

At the time, I was also working as a research assistant at a local heart institute and research center in Kansas City. This gave me a front row seat to the interplay of the business and medical consequences when the story first broke. Beyond the financial repercussions we were discussing in class, huge waves were being made in the medical community as well.

As news of the study spread, doctors became inundated with calls from worried patients. Some practitioners even admitted to taking their phones off the hook. "I'm just letting all my calls go to the answering machine," said Dr. Wulf Utian, executive director of the North American Menopause Society. "This is the biggest bombshell that ever hit in my 30-something years in the menopause area."

Medical professionals scrambled to respond to the news that estrogen replacement—once deemed the standard treatment for menopausal women—was suddenly something to fear.

The prevailing wisdom in 2001 had been the same for the last quarter-century: Once women begin menopause and start losing estrogen, taking systemic hormone replacements provides a safety net of positive effects and disease prevention. Hormone therapy cured hot flashes, kept the bones strong, helped skin stay healthy, bolstered a waning sex drive, and warded off heart disease and dementia. For some patients, estrogen therapy did carry a risk of breast cancer, but without a personal or immediate family history of the disease, it wasn't considered something to worry about.

The infamous study that would eventually disrupt the unchallenged use of hormone replacement for menopausal women was one of epic proportions. Beginning in the early 1990s, a drug trial for the study by the National Institutes of Health (NIH) enrolled more than 160,000 women in a multi-year comparison of hormone pills versus placebos. The study was scheduled to run until 2005. But as the results came back, investigators from the Women's Health Initiative (WHI) deemed the hormones too dangerous for the participants to even continue using through the remainder of the study. They had to abort the largest clinical trial ever conducted on women's health because participants who took certain combined hormones had a 26 percent increased chance of breast cancer—as well as a significantly higher risk of heart attack, stroke, and blood clots in the lungs—compared with those taking the placebo. Other parts of the same federal study later found that these drugs also actually increased the risk of dementia in a subset of participants age 65 and older.

This news impacted the lives of millions of women who relied on hormone replacement to ease the symptoms of menopause. Estrogen replacement was essentially considered a blessing to so many women who depended on it to help negate the hormonal upheaval. Press releases about the study induced such a panic that millions of women immediately decided to forgo the existing benefits of hormone replacement. While my classmates and I understood the study was exciting, none of us truly digested the shakeup it would cause across the medical community and the world.

Fifteen years later, the impact of this announcement continues to perplex patients and doctors regarding what sounds like a rather straight-forward question: Yes or no to estrogen replacement therapy?

One of the most consequential effects of menopause is depression. While some women will experience mood swings caused by hormonal shifts or may feel some symptoms of "the blues," about 20 percent of menopausal women will develop clinical depression. A study from the National Institute of Mental Health found that the risk of depression for menopausal women was 14 times higher than for women in premenopause.

This isn't a diagnosis to take lightly. Heather Chetwynd, described by her husband Robert as "a very lively and bubbly woman," suffered from severe depression as a result of menopause. She experienced significant mood swings on a daily basis. "Mostly," her husband recounted, "she would stare at the television. When I would talk to her, she would hear me without listening."

On a morning in March 2014, the 52-year-old mother of two started the day by spending time with her husband. "She seemed very happy and calm," he explained—the pair had just returned from Exmoor, where they'd been on a sightseeing trip together. But before Robert made it home from work that evening, Heather retreated to the back patio with one of her husband's shotguns and took her own life. Robert was shocked and devastated.

Though she had been prescribed antidepressants by her doctor, Heather did not like drugs and took the medication only sporadically. Because of her high blood pressure, she had been afraid to try hormone replacement therapy, wary of the many risks that had been brought to light in years prior.

Estrone sulfate, isolated from the urine of pregnant mares, was introduced in the early 1940s as Premarin by the pharmaceutical company Wyeth. It remained in use for the next three decades as a treatment for the symptoms of menopause and osteoporosis. Trouble started in the mid-1970s, when two studies published in the *New England Journal of Medicine* reported that taking estrogen therapy increased the risk of endometrial cancer by at least five times. Researchers found a direct correlation between the rise of estrogen use starting in the mid-1960s and the spike in endometrial cancer incidences. It's estimated that more than 15,000 cases of endometrial cancer were caused by estrogen replacements in 1971–1975 alone.

Some professional organizations even reported that this represented one of the largest epidemics of a disease caused by physician-administered treatments in history. The result was a precipitous decrease in estrogen use, with women who already used estrogen replacement reporting they were gripped in fear that they would soon fall victim to endometrial cancer themselves.

Then started the roller coaster. Relief came when another study debunked this negative reputation of estrogen. The mid-1990s saw the surge of several studies in reputed peer review journals reporting a protective effect of hormone drugs on heart health. Wyeth built a marketing campaign around its next estrogen drug, a new combination hormone called Prempro. This drug included another female hormone called progestin to keep estrogen from causing excessive cell growth in the uterine lining. Wyeth successfully repositioned menopausal hormone therapy as a preventive health choice that could help inhibit heart disease and other maladies.

Sales of Wyeth's hormone drugs peaked at about $2 billion in 2001, but the success didn't last long. In 2002, the year the WHI study was published, a woman by the name of Connie Barton came forward with news that she had taken Prempro from 1997 to 2002. She stopped taking the drug when she was diagnosed with breast cancer, which resulted in a mastectomy to remove her left breast. A storm of 13,000 women followed, collectively suing Wyeth with claims that after taking Prempro to prevent heart disease and dementia, they were later diagnosed with breast cancer or other diseases.

After the results of the 2002 study were published, Prempro's sales plummeted. By June 2012, Pfizer Inc., the world's largest drug-maker, said in a securities filing that it had paid close to $1 billion to resolve about 60 percent of the cases alleging its menopause drugs caused cancer in women. They paid an average of $150,000 per case.

The story of the hormone replacement saga doesn't end there. Researchers returned to the WHI study to examine post-intervention outcomes, and these findings surprised again. Data published in the *Journal of the American Medical Association* in 2011 indicated that certain women who used only estrogen during the original study did, in fact, have a markedly reduced risk for breast cancer and heart attacks.

Confused?

The results seemed logical enough until these studies began producing conflicting results depending on the type of hormone, administration methods, and ages of the patients receiving the therapy.

Today, physicians prescribe Premarin to women who have had hysterectomies and therefore are not at risk for endometrial cancer. Yet there is no clear consensus regarding the long-term effects of the hormone on health conditions like heart disease, dementia, and bone strength.

There are other instances in which a physician's recommendations fall into a gray area, such as if and when to check PSA (Prostate Specific Antigen) levels, ever-changing recommendations for PAP smears and mammograms, the necessity of ordering screening scans for lung cancers, and blood tests for some hormone disorders.

If the purpose of clinical studies is to bring doctors and patients to a point of standardized decision-making, how are we justifying the promise of this practice? To understand how the science of statistical studies changed the face of medicine and what we can learn from it, we have to go back to examine the basis upon which doctors used to make life-altering decisions and how patients came to trust this newfound approach.

CHAPTER 8

HOW MATHEMATICIANS CHANGED MEDICAL PRACTICE

> It is very important to reject every empirical process, and
> to complete the analysis, so that it shall not be necessary to
> derive from observations any but indispensable data.
>
> —PIERRE-SIMON LAPLACE, *TRAITÉ MÉCANIQUE CÉLESTE*
>
> Progress towards truth is impaired in the presence of an expert.
>
> —DAVID SACKETT, PIONEER IN EVIDENCE-BASED MEDICINE

British physician Richard Lower became the nucleus of the Royal Society in the 1660s when he demonstrated how shaking an open glass tube containing venous blood changed the dark purplish color to bright red as it mixed with air. As this happened right before the eyes of the audience, Lower categorically proved how venous blood becomes arterial. Then, via his methodical dissections, he traced the circulation of blood as it passed through the lungs and heart. Working like a chemist, he demonstrated how the blood in the test tube behaved like that in our body as it passed through the lungs, stating:

> That this red color is entirely due to the penetration of particles of air into the blood is quite clear from the fact that, while the blood becomes red throughout its mass in the lungs, when venous blood is collected in a vessel its surface takes on this scarlet color from exposure to air.

Although it's obvious that the blood in our bodies and blood in a test tube will not exhibit identical properties, the physiochemical activities in the human body were treated no differently than a set of chemical reactions studied in laboratories under controlled conditions. This crude approximation became a necessity in exploring the mechanisms of bodily functions without relying on myth and speculation.

Using controlled experiments, scientists started discovering several isolated biological processes that had until then remained obscure, such as blood circulation, digestion, respiration, and so on. After studying them independently, the goal of piecing together these various vital functions through additional experiments was set in motion. But physiologists soon realized that this exercise was uniquely challenging. While analyzing individual biological phenomena seemed straightforward, it became a formidable task for the human mind to interlink the various, dynamically changing biochemical processes within our bodies.

One such area was determining the appropriate dose of drug for a particular condition. For centuries, healers were used to dispensing drugs based on arbitrary estimates, sometimes by hunch, most often by accepted wisdom, and without any standard guidelines. As we started to understand how our bodies metabolize various drugs, we discovered that determining the appropriate dosage of a drug for an individual depends on many factors. These can include how fast it will dissolve in the stomach (or blood), its interaction with diet and other drugs, and how it's excreted from the body. We learned that if a drug is supplied in a form that dissolves too quickly or too slowly, it may yield an ineffective or toxic effect that can result in inadequate treatment or even death. Tracking and measuring a drug's impact at this level of complexity becomes an impossible task in biological experiments unless there is a method to incorporate these variables into a model that can analyze the conditions simultaneously.

Corresponding with the discovery of new biological mechanisms was the conception of newer methods to treat various illnesses. As new ideas were being introduced into medical practices, physicians desperately needed a tool that could evaluate the strength of evidence for or against that particular treatment. If such ambiguities weren't addressed, this budding science would have been left at risk of spiraling back down into the dark ages of metaphysical and speculative theories.

It was mathematicians who came to physicians' aid. The man whose theories would forever change the study of experimental medicine was the very same man who discovered the laws of gravity. Working as a professor at Trinity College, the celebrated seventeenth-century mathematician Isaac Newton was required to serve as a minister at the university's church. This was an obligation for all faculty members, despite Newton's total opposition to the rule. Like the sixteenth-century physician Michael Servetus (who was burnt on a pile of his own books for going against the idea of the Holy Trinity), Newton also did not believe in the doctrine of the triad of God, Son, and Holy Spirit.

Though he was dedicated to science, Newton owned 30 versions of the Bible and wrote more on theology than physics, astronomy, and mathematics combined. Newton strongly believed, through rigorous research of ancient theological treatises, that it was the third- and fourth-century Greek philosophers who incorporated the concept of the Trinity into theology. He also believed that the original idea had nothing to do with an all-powerful god. Unlike his predecessors, who were persecuted for their free-thinking, Newton was neither subdued nor ostracized by the orthodoxy. His life was spared not because of his popularity or the importance of his studies, but because religion was slowly beginning to loosen its tight grip on many areas of scientific exploration.

During his studies, Newton developed extensive methods by which to calculate the properties of fluctuating entities. He named his paper "Fluxion," which would later come to be known as calculus.[1] Another mathematician, German-born Gottfried Leibniz, also developed calculus independently but around the same time.

Until that time, if we wanted to study how two variables influenced each other, there was no quick way to intuitively interpret the dynamic interaction. Calculus opened the door for us, allowing us to observe the rates of changing functions such as time, force, mass, length, or temperature. The relationships between many quantifiable entities in nature could now be understood using these complex mathematical computations. This eventually became the language of experimentation.

. . .

Before the seventeenth century, the medical profession had no interest in the collection and analysis of data. They therefore also saw no value in using calculations in their treatments. It was not a physician or even a mathematician but a tradesman by the name of John Graunt who first utilized statistics in the medical field.

Even with no formal education, Graunt became fascinated with mortality statistics. He compiled a book based on his research of the Bills of Mortality, a collection of vital statistics about the citizens of

---

1   "Calculus," which in Latin means *small pebble*, was not introduced into mainstream mathematics until the seventeenth century. Until then, it was only applied to marketplace addition or subtraction.

London spanning over 70 years. Published in England in 1665, Graunt's book *Natural and Political Observations Mentioned in a following Index, and Made upon the Bills of Mortality* (referred to as *Observations*), illustrated the accounts that were kept as the number of London deaths rose from the plague, which killed one-fourth of England's population in the year 1625 alone.

Observations attempted to create a system to warn of the onset and spread of the plague, and it paved the way for the usefulness of data in medicine. Over the next 100 years, statistical thinking began to pervade every area of medicine, from research to policy. These influences came largely from outside healthcare. It was two mathematicians, Thomas Bayes and Pierre-Simon Laplace, who changed the face of medicine forever.

By the late 1700s, French mathematician and astronomer Pierre-Simon Laplace was adamant that statistics should be applied to the entire system of human knowledge, not just physics or chemistry. In regards to medicine, he believed that as the number of observations (data points) increased, the best treatments would manifest themselves.

Laplace was a creative genius. He reduced the study of planets to a series of differential equations, attesting that the motion of the planets and the sun could simply be explained by the laws of Newton. He asserted that by analyzing data alone, we could study everything from the macro-universe to the smallest atom.

His theory was based on simple yet profound logic he borrowed from his predecessors. He believed that since the world is too complicated for us to analyze all at once, progress can be made only if we study aspects of the universe separately. To do this, mathematical models that reproduce several features of one of these aspects, called physical theories, were constructed. Laplace firmly believed that we could construct a representation of reality through equations. The Pythagorean assertion of "All is number" ultimately found its fulfillment in Laplace's vision.

. . .

Laplace is most famous for his theory on the probability of events in nature. Commenting about his theory in his "Philosophical Essay on Probabilities" (1814), Laplace explained that "The theory of probabilities is basically common sense reduced to a calculus. It makes one estimate accurately what people feel by a sort of instinct, often without being able to give a reason for it."

For the first time in medicine, mathematics helped prove or disprove theories and tested the utility of different treatment options. It also bettered judgment by providing physicians with data for decision-making.

Laplace encouraged the use of statistical analysis to determine the validity of therapies. Prior to this, the common practice was to merely rely upon the passed-down experiences of senior physicians and anecdotal evidence, meaning there was no precise consistency across the field. Physicians felt that treatments were best chosen based on expert opinions rather than quantitative analysis. The introduction of statistics in medicine put this time-honored tradition to the test.

Physicists, mathematicians, and chemists began to share their thoughts and discoveries within their distinctive fields in professional societies to mutually advance their studies. Often, though, physicians didn't identify themselves as part of the scientific movement. Practitioners of this profession justified their aloofness, touting a long-held conviction that biology was too complicated and individualistic to be reduced to the general application of simple laws. It took significant persuasion for physicians to become an intricate part of the network of sciences.

Famous physicians like Pierre-Jean-Georges Cabanis (1757–1808) attempted to establish best practices for the proper professional approach toward diagnostic dilemmas in the final decades of the century. The consensus was that physicians should be able to judge individual patients based on their uniqueness rather than on quantitative assessments. Cabanis dismissed quantitative reasoning as a distraction and regarded medicine as more of an art than a science. There were few outliers to these generally established practices.

. . .

One prominent physician, Pierre-Charles Alexandre Louis (1787–1872), believed that applying analytical methods to therapeutic practices enabled better judgment and the avoidance of common misconceptions. Instead of relying on experience alone, his method involved meticulous observation and record-keeping, analysis of multiple cases, and verification through autopsies. Louis believed that through the power of statistics, all medical practitioners could arrive at consistent outcomes.

And Louis was right. For the first time in the practice of medicine, a statistical study was used to discredit a medical practice that needed to be subdued because of extravagant claims its creator was making without any factual basis. That creator was Franz Mesmer.

Mesmer was a German physician who claimed the human body contained a "psychic ether," a magnetic substance. In his 1774 treatise, he claimed that magnetism was the cause for some diseases, and therefore these diseases should be treated by way of controlling the individual's energy. Mesmer passionately favored the use of magnetism for treating nervous disorders, which he termed "animal magnetism."

Mesmer's popularity grew quickly, and he published hundreds of papers on animal magnetism as his followers rapidly proliferated. But Mesmer's popularity also triggered his downfall. Animal magnetism became such a craze that it drew the attention of the king. In 1784, having grown suspicious of the grandiose claims of the new practice, France's King Louis XVI appointed Benjamin Franklin to lead a commission of inquiry into Mesmer's practice.

The committee consisted of distinguished members of the scientific community and was tasked with investigating the medical claims of Mesmer's theory. The goal of the study was to assess whether the reported results of this healing method were real or a sort of placebo effect,[2] called then an "illness of the mind." The study involved telling blindfolded people that they were either receiving or not receiving magnetism and then assessing their response to the treatment. The results proved what the commission already suspected: Those who were told they received magnetism when they actually did not still claimed to experience the effects of the treatment. This study essentially put an end to the claims of mesmerism as a therapeutic option. Mesmer, disgraced as a charlatan, was driven into exile after the investigations.

Additional studies to legitimize the utility of medical practices followed suit. The pinnacle was reached when one study questioned the usefulness of bloodletting, the proverbial practice that had gone unchallenged for nearly 19 centuries. In the aftermath of the French Revolution, Parisian doctor François Joseph Victor Broussais (1772–1838) claimed that all fevers had the same origin: They were manifestations of inflamed organs. Accordingly, leeches were applied to the surface of the body corresponding to the site of the inflammation, and the resultant bloodletting was deemed an efficient treatment. Such theories were highly regarded by contemporary French physicians. This influence can be assessed using an economic measure: In 1825, France exported 10 million leeches, and by 1833, they imported 40 million more.

Unsatisfied with the lack of evidence to support the common practice of bloodletting, Louis conducted a study of typhoid fever. He collected data for five years in the 1800s to study the efficacy of the practice. Among 52 fatal cases, he observed that 75 percent had undergone

---

2   Doctors, until the nineteenth century, routinely used "placebos" (literally meaning *to please* in Latin) as part of their treatments.

bloodletting. The results perplexed fellow physicians. Louis's numerical analysis showed that bloodletting increased, rather than decreased, mortality. He used the same method to study the efficacy of bloodletting in the treatment of pneumonitis and tonsillitis and found no evidence to support its ability to treat these illnesses either. He encouraged fellow physicians to utilize quantitative analysis rather than blindly follow unproven theories. His analysis was practically heretical to the medical community, but to Louis, assumptions meant nothing. Facts were facts, and they were the only key to any truth, including in medicine.

At last, the prospect of developing methods to validate a therapy aided by the use of mathematical models seemed bright. But it would take well over another century to convince the medical profession to incorporate statistical methods in their practice.

. . .

In the late 1830s, urologist Jean Civiale (1792–1867) discovered a new bloodless method for removing bladder stones. To prove that his method was better than the current practice, he published the comparative rates of deaths from both the traditional surgical procedure and his new method, which he called lithotrity. The death rate of the old procedure was 22 percent, while the death rate for lithotrity fell to a mere 2 percent.

These convincing results led the Paris Academics of Science and Medicine to establish a commission led by mathematician Simeon-Denis Poission and physician François Double. Double was devastated by the inclusion of a mathematician in the organization, stating that it was inappropriate to elevate the "human spirit to the statistical certainty that you can find in astronomy."

Double believed that progress in medicine was possible only by logic and intuition, and that numerical analysis had no place. He even went so far as to comment that statistical models would reduce the doctor to "a shoemaker who, after having measured the feet of a thousand, persisted in fitting everyone on the basis of the imaginary model."

Many held stubbornly to the belief that mathematics was unfit to analyze therapeutic practices. The medical community, for instance, didn't even realize that postpartum mothers in the doctors' wards of Vienna General Hospital's First Obstetrical Clinic had a mortality rate of a whopping 35 percent until the Hungarian physician Ignaz Philipp Semmelweis measured it in 1847. To everyone's surprise, he discovered that doctors' wards had mortality rates three times as high as those of midwives. His finding that hand washing was able to reduce mortality rates to below 1 percent had already been published, but the medical community had not yet embraced the practice, and Semmelweis's observations were rejected. In fact, some doctors even took offense to the idea that they needed to sanitize before attending to patients. But sticking to these antiquated, flawed practices had terrible consequences: Many newborns were left motherless.

Nevertheless, this objective approach started to capture the attention of a few doctors. In 1865, as the 38-year-old Joseph Lister walked the wards of his Glasgow hospital, he was unable to escape the rotten stench of putrefying flesh—a scent that would nauseate even the most unstirred minds. The outcomes of many surgeries at this time were a pitiable state of affairs.

A surgeon's routine was like nothing we'd allow for today. Surgical garb was a point of pride and attested to these doctors' busy practices. Proof of their hard work was recognized by coats stiffened with blood and pus, the threaded needles secured to the buttonholes. The operating room was equipped with sinks adorned with brass taps; marble-topped tables for bottles, towels, and used sponges; a pail of sand to overlay sticky blood on the floorboards; wooden boxes with sawdust to dispose of amputated limbs; and hot iron rods used to cauterize bleeding wounds. Mortality rates were so high that operating rooms were built next to hospitals' mortuaries.

Lister observed that from 1864 to 1866, the average mortality rate for all surgical procedures performed at the University of Edinburgh was 46 percent. The prevailing theory blamed polluted air for the fatalities, but no one really knew how to control the ravage this caused. Influenced by French chemist Louis Pasteur[3] and his germ theory, Lister believed it was microbes carried in the air that caused diseases to spread in operating rooms. As a result, he developed a machine to pump a fine mist of carbolic acid into the operating room during surgeries. After the introduction of Lister's antiseptic methods, the mortality rate for all surgical procedures performed from 1867–70 fell to 15 percent. Lister published these findings of his groundbreaking work with antiseptic surgery in 1870.

While Louis Pasteur and Robert Koch developed the germ theory of disease, it was Lister who was instrumental in implementing the practical application of the theory relating to hygienic surgical practices and markedly decreasing the spread of disease during procedures as a result. The division of surgical history into pre- and post-Listerian eras speaks volumes about his impact on fighting infections. But without statistical confirmation of the dramatic drop in mortality, Lister could not have convinced his colleagues to consider his antiseptic theory or his approach to surgical sanitation.

While these improvements were starting to alter the landscape of medicine, resistance from physicians was far more prevalent than a willingness to adopt new practices. But not for long.

---

3   Pasteur was responsible for disproving the archaic doctrine of *spontaneous generation*, the belief that life could come from nonliving things, such as mice from corn, flies from bovine manure, and maggots from rotting meat. Pasteur met intense opposition by the entire religio-medical establishment, because of his opposition to the unchallenged doctrine laid by the ancients dating back to Aristotle. It was only his persistence and sound experimental and analytical procedures that finally compelled most biological and medical scientists to discard the long-held belief. (*Men of Science-Men of God* by Henry Morris, ISBN 0-89051-080-6)

. . .

Twenty-seven-year-old Karl Pearson was no ordinary mathematician. As the newly appointed professor of mathematics at University College London, he believed he could explain almost everything about "plants, animals, and men" through the application of statistics. "There is no sphere of inquiry which lies outside the legitimate field of science," he wrote in his acclaimed book on statistics, cleverly titled *The Grammar of Science*. He developed statistical methodology and attempted to convince the world that this was the next-best way to analyze problems related to biology. His theory of statistical relevancy found few audiences, though. The Royal Society rejected his papers, as biologists found it preposterous for mathematicians to interfere in their space.

. . .

The medical profession was divided on the use of statistical methodology. Those who viewed medicine as an "art" couldn't digest the idea of crunching numbers to study human biology. Others argued that medicine was a "science" and saw statistics as a means for more objective observation. It would be a student of Pearson's who would go on to evoke massive appeal to statistics in medicine.

Major Greenwood, perhaps Pearson's most devoted follower, was a trained doctor in London in 1905. He chose to study under Pearson despite the obvious financial shortcomings of being a statistician. Pearson had the opportunity to turn Greenwood into the first medical statistician and he took full advantage, training him into a numerical wizard who could fully apply statistical methodology to medical practices.

Greenwood's persistence paid off. He was soon appointed the head of the newly established Department of Statistics at the Lister Institute of Preventive Medicine in London. His reputation spread across the

Atlantic, and he began to work with American counterparts to investigate the application of mathematics in the study of human disease. His methods were slowly gaining popularity in the most elite inner circles.

The medical community began to agree that studying statistics was a vital part of training to be a physician, as it ensured that medicine was grounded in science. Greenwood managed to influence some of the young physicians of the time, but it was one of his apprentices—a non-physician by the name of Austin Bradford Hill—who would go on to become the primary driver of using standardized research studies to evaluate the effectiveness and safety of medical devices or drugs. Today, these are known as clinical trials.

Hill supervised a remarkable study with an impressive degree of planning and execution. The clinical trial sought to tackle a prevalent disease with high mortality rates: pulmonary tuberculosis (TB). The British Medical Council decided to test the use of streptomycin in the treatment of tuberculosis under Hill's supervision. Patients were gathered from several geographical centers and randomly assigned to one of two treatment arms: either streptomycin plus bed-rest or bed-rest alone (the placebo). Each patient's chest X-ray was independently reviewed by two radiologists and a clinician. The results would forever change the fate of mycobacterium, the microbe that causes TB. The study proved that patient survival improved significantly with the use of streptomycin.

In writing about his experiences during the design of this large-scale clinical trial in "Memories of the British Streptomycin Trial in Tuberculosis—The First Randomized Clinical Trial," Hill shared:

> The concepts of "randomization" and "random sampling numbers" are slightly odd to the layman, or, for that matter, the lay doctor, when it comes to statistics. I thought it would be better to get doctors to walk first, before I tried to get them to run.

Hill was a trailblazer, convincing the medical community to accept the utility of statistics on a massive scale in therapeutics. He was also a visionary. He was a firm believer that those in medicine should not be limited to curing the sick, but also had a responsibility to advance the understanding of health and diseases. This meant that doctors should take up research as a career in addition to their clinical practice. By doing so, he believed that doctors could incorporate the latest scientific knowledge into medical treatments.

Hill was also lucky. The timing was perfect, as new and potent drugs were being industrially produced in the post-war era. He was able to rally supporters for the use of statistical methods to study the efficacy of newly discovered drugs on humans, a concept that had never before been considered.

Prior to World War II, research was very small scale and generally consisted of a few doctors working independently using their own patients, families, and neighbors as subjects. Most of these studies were conducted for immediate, self-serving purposes, such as to find a treatment plan for a particular case. In the past, a few scientists—like Joseph Lister and his work on antisepsis—proved useful, but the small scope of the research typically didn't have much impact on the overall practice of medicine.

It was Hill's experiments in the 1940s that laid the groundwork for larger studies in which both the insight of physicians and the statistical design of professional statisticians were combined. Laplace's vision of using calculus and statistics to explain biological phenomena was finally actualized.

The basic model of statistical methodology was now universally applied to almost every aspect of medicine. Select a topic to investigate, observe and measure the phenomenon, collect data, translate it into equations to be solved and interpreted, and then draw a conclusion. It was working. Larger and larger populations were put to the test by researchers undertaking some of the most expensive experiments in history.

In 1954, a study was performed on the effectiveness of the Salk vaccine as protection against paralysis or death from polio. With the annual incidence rate of polio at about 1 in 2,000, the medical community was desperate for a cure. Ethically, it was a struggle to convince parents to allow their children to be randomized into the placebo group, but ultimately two million children participated, costing more than five million dollars. It was the largest and most expensive study of the time. It also changed the world as we knew it.

The Salk vaccine proved effective.

Once the methodology gained such large-scale exposure, the debate to include statistical reasoning in medicine became a public-policy issue, no longer controlled by inner circles of physicians. With this shift, the use of computation and statistical reasoning became the norm, leading to large-scale randomized controlled trials like the WHI study on estrogen replacement therapy published in 2002.

The application of statistics to medicine changed the game across every arena of the field. Microbiologists, for instance, began using calculus to determine the exact rate of growth in a bacterial culture when different variables such as temperature, moisture, and food source were altered. Statistical analysis of this research helped assess the growth curves of different bacterial strains and compared the effectiveness of different antibiotics on these cultures, which aided in the discovery of potent new antibiotics.

Another field that relies on statistics is epidemiology, the study of the spread of infectious disease. Applying quantitative reasoning, we've been able to determine the rate of spread of disease and the extent of spread in populations. This is especially important because rates of infection and recovery change over time, so disease control measures must also change accordingly to respond to new disease patterns as they evolve.

The use of statistics in healthcare has not only provided an understanding of individual health but has also continued to provide key indicators of the health of entire nations and even the world as a whole. By truly understanding the health of different populations, we've been able to promote necessary cultural shifts and establish appropriate practices that cater to the unique needs of a specific region. Physicians have been able to better track emerging threats like epidemics, such as helping us mitigate the flu pandemic each year.

. . .

Statistical methods radically transformed the doctor's practice. Individual opinions and anecdotal evidence were relegated as the least reliable form of information. This was a 180-degree turn from medicine's earlier history, when these were the most valid references. Randomized controlled trials were elevated to the gold standard, and all physicians were expected to abide. It is now accepted that virtually no drug, no surgical therapy, and no diagnostic test can enter clinical practice without demonstration of its efficacy in clinical trials.

It painstakingly took nearly 200 years to develop this tool to help the medical community. The use of statistics in medical practice was finally able to deliver the profession from deep-rooted metaphysical theorists and unify physicians into a cohesive group of like-minded thinkers.

In their work, doctors and researchers have typically been careful to frame the outcomes of statistical evidence within the context of a particular situation. But when communicated to the public, these same results often get passed along in terms that are more black and white. Headlines blast sensational news that a medication has been found to be completely safe or unsafe, and panic ensues as a result. Like most findings in the medical world, though, the issue of the safety of a drug—like hormone replacement therapy for menopause—is far more nuanced. The decision to take estrogen supplements falls along a spectrum of pros and cons, a teeter of benefits one has to weigh against potential risks. The science of statistics allows for the development of general guidelines, and then the "art" of medicine provides for the individualization of that generality.

CHAPTER 9

THE OBSESSION WITH MEASURING THE HUMAN BODY

Measure what can be measured, and make measurable what cannot be measured.

—GALILEO GALILEI

We are but waterproof bags of electrically charged chemicals, which one day befall a power failure.

—RICHARD GORDON, *THE ALARMING HISTORY OF MEDICINE*

In May of 2013, in the middle of a 14-hour flight from Chicago to New Delhi, I heard an overhead announcement in a voice rattled with anxiety: "Any doctor on board, please attend to a sick person." I squeezed past my seatmate into the narrow aisle where a pale, middle-aged man sat several rows back.

When I asked him what was wrong, the man spoke sluggishly and complained of dizziness. I checked to make sure he was breathing without difficulty and was relieved to find that he was. But I tensed when I felt only a feeble pulse strike against my fingers through the cold, clammy skin of his wrist.

The man's wife stood next to him, squeezing her fingers hard into the back of the seat. I kept my voice measured and calm as I spoke to her. After a quick survey of the man, I asked, "Have there been any recent major medical issues?" I suggested a few: "Heart disease, stroke, high blood pressure, diabetes, anything like that?" and braced for her response.

"He suffered a heart attack two years ago," she explained. The man had a stent in his heart. Immediately, I went on high alert. On a typical day at the hospital where I work, I'm used to ordering tests, reviewing blood work, and measuring various bodily functions. This information is always instantly at my disposal. But there I was, 30,000 feet in the air, searching for clues about what's going on inside the body of this hapless person in front of me as the flight attendant hurried to locate an emergency medical kit.

The few minutes that passed felt like an eternity, but finally I was handed a shabby stethoscope missing an ear piece and a dilapidated blood-pressure monitor. The pulse I'd been feeling with my own fingers was still faint. My stomach dropped when I realized the blood-pressure monitor was broken. I attempted to maintain my confidence, but my own palms were sweating now as I realized the remaining contents of the airplane's emergency medical kit were of no use to me—a few bandages and alcohol wipes, but no basic equipment such as a blood sugar meter or even a thermometer.

I was on board one of the most marvelous creations of the human mind—the airplane—and I felt helpless. A host of questions ran through my mind. *What if he's having a stroke? What's my plan if this is, indeed, a heart attack? If he's bleeding internally from a ruptured aorta, what can I do to maintain his blood pressure until we land? What if, what if, what if.*

Without instruments to measure the most basic vital parameters such as blood sugar or blood pressure, I had to assemble the meager clues available to me and then rely on my own experience and intuition to make an educated guess. "Does he have a blood sugar problem?" I asked.

"No," his wife said, "but sometimes he feels dizzy if he misses a meal." In the family's rush to make their flight that morning, the man had skipped breakfast.

I didn't want to cause pandemonium, but I also didn't want to spread false hope. Though I couldn't be certain, my gut told me it wasn't his heart. I reassured the man's family and the rest of the flight staff that I didn't think the man was in mortal danger. I noticed a sigh of relief on the flight captain's face while he looked up to me as I comforted the crowd. But without the aid of technology, tests, or instruments, only I knew how powerless I felt. I took a deep breath and reminded myself of my role in this situation. There are two timeless precepts of the medical profession that never change: First, do whatever it takes to reassure and comfort the sick. Second, do my best to identify the sickness and relieve the individual's distress.

Experience and a bit of luck pointed me toward an educated guess that my patient's dizziness might be caused by low blood sugar. I asked the flight attendant for orange juice and instructed the man to slowly swallow down two cups of it. This was the least and the best I could offer in that situation. After the man finished the drink, I asked his row-mates to give up their seats so he could lie down.

Luckily, within a few minutes his color returned and his pulse felt stronger. When he started talking again, the rest of us on board shared a feeling of immense relief. I ran into the man again after we exited the flight in New Delhi, and by this time, he said he was feeling just fine.

This experience left me thinking about the power of measurement. For a physician, the key indicators used to assess a patient's health are the vital parameters we're able to measure: heart rate, respiratory rate, temperature, blood pressure, and so on. Without measurements, a doctor's ability to accurately assess a patient becomes severely limited.

In the process of quantification of almost all aspects of human biology, doctors make systematic observations as a valid way of building knowledge about a patient's health in order to then prognosticate the efficacy of treatments. Doctors are taught to think of a patient's health in terms of numbers. A typical doctor's visit ends by giving a patient a set of goals to meet: lowered cholesterol, controlled blood pressure or heart rate, a target blood sugar, or a measured thyroid or PSA level.

For centuries, healers depended solely on patients' narratives, through which they would guess what was wrong. It wasn't until the seventeenth century that quantification became the primary factor in the study of human biology. This approach created a perceptual shift in how physicians "see" patients—using vital parameters, which are nothing but numbers—as a critical means to understanding and assessing one's health.

. . .

The first major contribution that changed the fate of medical practice was the pendulum clock, invented in 1656 by Dutch mathematician Christiaan Huygens. For 3,000 years, we'd used the sundial to mark the passage of time, but as civilizations grew, so did the need for more precise timekeeping. It wasn't until the swinging pendulum was made available for public use in the eighteenth century that we divided day and night into regular and shorter periods of time.

With this invention, many aspects of human biology could be recorded in precise intervals. Counting how fast we breathe and how briskly our hearts beat per minute became the universal measure of our vital functions.

Next, we tackled body temperature. Without a standard scale, records of body temperature were educated guesses. Fever, for instance, was determined by a doctor placing his or her palm against a patient's forehead.

The thermometer changed this practice. It's one of the best illustrations of the movement toward quantification—an essential dimension of the mathematization of nature. It took well over a century of tough grind to standardize this method. Finally, in 1868, Carl Wunderlich conducted a study using his foot-long thermometer in which he painstakingly measured the axillary temperature of 25,000 patients on multiple visits for a total of over one million readings in all. Based on his analysis, he was able to establish a range for normal temperature, which is 36.3–37.5 °C. Any temperature outside of this range suggested an internal disturbance. This was a critical discovery. The impact was immediate, allowing a new way for doctors to look for the presence of an illness or infection.

Unlike our long-standing fascination with temperature and time, determining blood pressure didn't arouse the same curiosity from the medical community for quite some time. Despite the pervasive loss of blood through bloodletting as a treatment for many ailments, it wasn't until Stephan Hales's experiments in the middle of the eighteenth century that physicians' interest in this measurement grew. In 1727, Hales was the first to determine arterial blood pressure when he measured the rise in a column of blood in a glass tube inserted into an artery. It was another century before the practice moved from the lab to the clinic, thanks to Jean Léonard Marie Poiseuille and his doctoral dissertation on the use of the mercury manometer for measuring blood pressure. His work earned him the Gold Medal of the Royal Academy of Medicine in 1828.

Because of his experiments on the flow of human blood in narrow tubes, Poiseuille was famously called the first "physician-physicist." Further, vigorous development of this technique throughout the latter half of the nineteenth century allowed blood pressure to finally attain distinction as one of the most important metrics of life. The reputation for this shift is so revered in the medical community that some consider the measurement of blood pressure to be more impactful than the discovery of blood itself.

. . .

Quantification became the driving force behind the modern scientist's quest to reduce every entity to its simplest and most fundamental indivisible, measurable unit. The word "atom" was originally used as a metaphor. Derived from Greek, "a-tomos" means *not-cuttable*, as in, *that which cannot be cut further*—the building block of all matter. By applying this approach, every aspect of nature was sliced and probed to its most basic level: for light, photons; for biology, the cell; for temperature, degrees Celsius; for length, the meter; for sound, the decibel.

Physicians applied these metrics liberally to the human body, which gave them the ability to measure and experiment. Three centuries of perseverance to standardize these methods in medicine paid off. Physicians were enabled to distinguish a normal biological process from an abnormal one. They were also empowered with a numerical designation as a universal method of communication that crossed geographical and language boundaries.[1]

Scientists not only came to create uniform methods to measure many aspects of the biological world, they also cataloged all known living entities. Physician-turned-botanist Carl Linnaeus essentially immortalized Latin as the universal language of science by giving each species two-word Latin names through a systematic method of identification. He arranged everything in the living world into a particular order—first

---

1 Musicians had already conceived this idea centuries prior. They divided the sound into smaller, more digestible pieces, and gave them notations so that they could capture the naturally-produced vibrations from vocal cords into different combinations of music. Eventually, they applied this notation to instruments like flute and violin. After a while, when technology allowed artificial production of sound, they applied the notations to synthesizers to make more music. Musical notation is nothing but a method of slicing the whole into pieces so that they can be reproduced and rearranged.

by a kingdom and class, then by the subdivisions of genus and species. In the wake of Linnaeus's work, biologists across the world were able to specify all living things in the same language.

Linnaeus forever changed humankind's place in nature by being the first person to include humans in the biological scheme alongside animals and plants. The decision to classify humans as Homo sapiens was met with considerable resistance from theological circles at the time. In a letter to a colleague in 1747, Linnaeus wrote: "If I were to call man ape or vice versa, I should bring down all the theologians on my head. But perhaps I should still do it according to the rules of the science." Despite disagreeing with popular theists, Linnaeus, being a religious man, believed that he was simply uncovering "God's handiwork" through his classification of nature.

. . .

Our quest to divide, classify, and measure every aspect of life's processes even stretched to the study of our intellect. George Boole believed that human logic could be quantified, and he dedicated his life to developing a "science of intellectual powers" of the mind. He believed that thinking and reasoning could be understood by applying laws of mathematics.

Also a religious man, Boole had a mystical vision at the age of 17 in which he felt God called him to develop theories about how the mind processed thoughts. He decided that mathematics would serve as the perfect medium for this purpose. He went on to create mathematical models "to unfold the secret laws" and relations of those high faculties of thought by which perceptive knowledge of the world and of ourselves is attained. He designed calculations to investigate the fundamental laws of the operations of the mind by which reasoning was performed. In his 1847 essay "Mathematical Analysis of Logic," he applied algebra to the deduction of logical problems and simplified the world to basic statements that had either yes or no answers. This opened a pathway to a new science of binary arithmetic in which all operations were expressed as either 0 or 1. More than a century later, this same expression would be applied to electrical switching circuits and computer language.

When it came to studying emotions, we initially ran into some difficulties applying experimental testing to our behavior. We first needed to develop a method to quantify human behavior.

Just like neurology was the study of the brain and nerves, psychology was emerging as the study of the mind. But there was a formidable hurdle to establish this as a separate discipline of medicine. Psychology was a part of philosophy that didn't provide a meaningful process for measurement of the ineffable human mind, which is without dimension or weight. It became necessary for psychologists to be able to understand the human mind through a more deliberate process of observation and quantification. Prior to the eighteenth century, the basic belief in European academia was that psychology as a science would never come to fruition. The only solution was to divorce psychology from philosophy and allow it to evolve as a separate discipline.

This separation pushed philosophers away from healing traditions and eventually made mainstream philosophy a thing of the past. The modern-day translation of philosopher is now simply *a deep thinker*.

While philosophy is based on reason, psychology as we know it today was founded on theories subjected to proof, a far cry from the ancient Greek root of "psychology," which literally translated to *the discourse of the soul*. The primary objective of a psychologist was to record and analyze sensations and thoughts by the same means a chemist used when assessing compounds. With the prominence of psychology, a progressive theory was born that consciousness could be broken down into various measurable aspects. The method of grouping and finding patterns was accomplished through quantified laboratory observation. Everything had to be anchored in evidence.

This method laid the foundation for future experiments on human emotions for the next two centuries. By the twentieth century, psychologists inferred that mental activities could be studied by recording measurable properties in our bodies. Mental stress, for instance, could be quantified by checking levels of stress hormones in the blood. Another modern example would be utilizing functional MRIs of the brain to study emotions.

Applying this approach, we explained emotions as a manifestation of chemical signaling: Love hormones, for example, were nothing more than the result of neurotransmitters like dopamine and oxytocin fueling pair bonding. Scientists were even able to show proof: If oxytocin receptors were blocked, the pair-bonding response was cut off.

They went on to map the areas responsible for love and desire in the brain, and then researchers dug deeper. They found that the blood levels of specific chemicals were significantly higher in couples who had just fallen in love. Certain molecules apparently played an important role in the social chemistry of humans, or at least in the phenomenon known as "love at first sight." Scientists declared these results were a confirmation of love's scientific basis. The experiences that define who we are could now be explained as neurochemical exchanges in our biomechanical workshop.

And after this, we went further still. Evolutionary scientists announced that they could explain even the most elusive of all human attributes. They vouched that parental love was merely nature's way of duping us into perpetuating our genes. The alchemy of bonding, they asserted, was simply acting out an aeon-old evolutionary script inked in our DNA. Sentiments such as empathy and altruism were reduced to nothing but the products of natural selection. The same went for intellect. Scientists further claimed to have identified where intelligence and problem-solving areas resided in the brain and set out to test their theories.

Experimental studies took much of the lure of the unknown from our exalted emotional responses. With such an approach, nearly all conceivable human expression was subjected to measurement. For abstract emotional aspects like happiness and pain, self-reporting scales were assigned. Psychometric scales for subjective well-being were created to measure happiness. Likewise, a pain scale (typically marked within a range of 1–10) was developed.

With such uncanny ingenuity, we've concluded that almost every aspect of the human mind can be explored by scientific methods. Scientists have provided insight into the psychological world, which, by convention, forbids entry. In body and mind, we found ourselves wholly within the jurisdiction of experimental study.

. . .

A renewed worldview emerged from the scientific revolution: If the human body is seen as a sort of machine, then searching for parallels between it and the indefinable concept of the soul is pointless. Since the adoption of this newfound outlook, spiritual beliefs have become a personal matter that have no place in the study of science. Many who believed in the existence of a soul sought alternative ways to represent this concept that didn't conflict with the emerging science. Every aspect of study was secularized for one goal: freedom of thought.

This unemotional, purely objective approach meant philosophers and scientists no longer spoke a common language. Until this time, it was common to instill metaphysical and theistic overtones into scientific writings. This interesting artistic overlay provided a poetic nuance to the descriptions of scientific topics.

It was toward the end of the Renaissance that the style of scientific writing we know today was first introduced. Medical research papers are dry, devoid of rhyme and ode, and full of complicated, technical language, like instruction manuals describing the workings of a machine. As physician Sir Thomas Browne wrote, "All deductions from metaphors, parables, allegories became bereft of force. Only real and rigid interpretations had the power to convince." The influential thinkers of the seventeenth century forever changed the sentiment of physicians—medicine was to become "a soul-less" profession, no different than any other field of science.

The theories of the past (which believed our health is the result of a balance of humors and that nature serves as the ultimate authority) were to be replaced by the theory that bodily functions should be explored using experiments in laboratories.

For clinicians, this move essentially meant casting aside 2,000 years of wisdom in favor of a new method.

As a result, practitioners of scientific medicine underwent a radical makeover. It worked. By leaving behind the subjective idealism, doctors gained extraordinary new insights about bodily functions. In this metamorphosis, doctors, albeit reluctantly, disposed themselves of many elements that had defined their profession from the beginning of time. The result: no more metaphysics, no more cherished beliefs, and no more mysticism.

The vision of Hippocrates to separate the physician from the philosopher and priest was finally actualized. The medicine man became the person of science, his priesthood relinquished. Simultaneously, the authority and expertise of curing illnesses unconditionally shifted from the priest to the physician.

The physician was stripped of his robes and dressed in a white coat, removing the artist's persona and ridding the lineage that had dominated the profession for centuries. Old taboos were washed away and a new healer emerged.

The Evolution of Medicine
—From Gods to Genes

The priest-physician of the ancient age believed that disease was an affliction from the angered gods. Later, pre-medieval healers thought that disease was a result of a person "lacking in spirit." This ideology was replaced by the belief that illness was the result of an imbalance of humors, a theory that reigned for approximately 23 centuries. This was followed by the current notion that illness is localized to organs: this concept was the birth of disease-centered medicine. It took millennia to arrive at this model of understanding illness. This is now replaced by genomic medicine, based on the evidence that disease is a result of an aberration in one or more genes. Treatment involves therapies aimed at genes, not just at the afflicted organs. We are currently experiencing the birth of genomic medicine and the future version of the modern doctor.

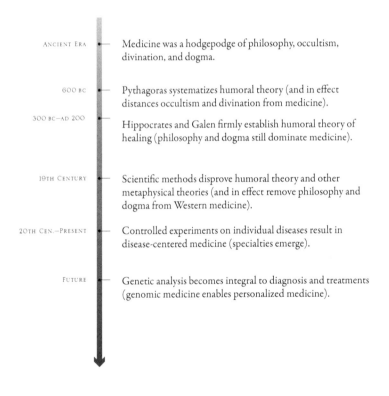

ANCIENT ERA — Medicine was a hodgepodge of philosophy, occultism, divination, and dogma.

600 BC — Pythagoras systematizes humoral theory (and in effect distances occultism and divination from medicine).

300 BC–AD 200 — Hippocrates and Galen firmly establish humoral theory of healing (philosophy and dogma still dominate medicine).

19TH CENTURY — Scientific methods disprove humoral theory and other metaphysical theories (and in effect remove philosophy and dogma from Western medicine).

20TH CEN.–PRESENT — Controlled experiments on individual diseases result in disease-centered medicine (specialties emerge).

FUTURE — Genetic analysis becomes integral to diagnosis and treatments (genomic medicine enables personalized medicine).

PART FOUR

THE BIG SHIFT

"Tactfully built into physicians' training is the ability for them to move from *feeling more, thinking less* to *feeling less, thinking more*."

CHAPTER 10

HOW THE HEART LOST ITS ESTEEMED POSITION

> Our heart always transcends us.
>
> —RAINER MARIA RILKE

"All clear. One. Two. Three. Shock!"

For 10 years, I've been running Code Blue, a term indicating the emergency situation in hospitals that requires attempting to revive a crashing patient. Nerve-racking and intense, the process is always challenging. Perfecting the art of staying calm in the midst of the storm is something doctors strive to attain constantly, no matter how experienced they may be.

The rush to bring back a vanished pulse, however, is a rather recent phenomenon; it's only about a century old in the medical profession. Physicians in antiquity were under much less pressure, or at least very different kinds of pressure, because they neither knew what happened to our body during cardiac arrest nor did they have the life-saving tools necessary to tend to the situation when it occurred. The prevailing belief, described in a physician's quote from 1890, was that "we are powerless against paralysis of the circulation." And for centuries, there were simply no effective means by which to revive a patient.

Physicians relied instead on the customary cure-all practices of the time: herbs, bloodletting, and incantations. Society was accustomed to the limited treatments a medicine man could provide and accepted the likely outcomes of either a quick death or, if they happened to survive, significant disability.

As an intern in the ICU of a community hospital, the night of my first Code Blue was harrowing. I raced to the patient's room after the call and was met with a frenzy of staff. I could hear the echo of my pulse thudding in my ears until it was replaced with the harsh beeping of equipment. The tension of the waiting staff felt like something palpable I had to push myself through as I crossed the threshold. As the house doctor assigned to codes that night, I was expected to take control of the situation and guide the team through the hopeful revival of the patient.

A nurse brought me up to speed as I entered: "56-year-old man became unresponsive after the nurse-aid put him to bed following lunch. She heard the patient choking just before he became listless."

I watched and heard everything around me, but there was also a marked distance—I didn't register much. I doubt I was alone in feeling this way. Each person on our team, tasked with a lifesaving purpose, was more supercharged than the next. A respiratory therapist handled an oxygen bag, pushing air into the middle-aged man's chest; one nurse administered IV meds while another performed chest compressions.

In the farthest corners of the room, medical students huddled among the comfort of their clan, observing in order to learn from the experience. Unlike the classroom, this lesson can be as intense and frenzying as watching a high-intensity sport. But unlike a game of football, which relies on the probability of error and defeat to stir us, a code situation can't tolerate missteps. This life-or-death setting does share one commonality with a vivacious game, however: the delicate teetering between skill and chance. The portion requiring skill involves the ability to manage randomness and master emotional reactions to unforeseen snags.

As more bodies circulated in and out to assist, I processed through a tunnel of focus—my own silent movie. The moment can only be classified as surreal. The patient had no pulse, but my own seemed to have tripled in speed. The monitor showed ventricular fibrillation, a malignant and life-threatening electrical rhythm of the heart.

The actions taking place around me appeared to speed up, yet I was wading through the room in slow motion. Before me was a complex puzzle to solve, one I'd been learning and training for, but in the moment of need, everything I thought I knew suddenly disappeared from my memory, as if someone had just pulled the power cord from the wall.

More supplies were requested. More fluids and drugs were administered. I stood at the end of the table, tapping my fingers nervously, watching. Adrenaline charging through my vessels; I took a step toward the patient. My face flushed and my eyes subtly twitched. I hadn't yet developed the knack of hiding my unease.

My senior resident, like a godsend, appeared in the room just then. Placing himself next to me, he whispered, "Check to see if the patient has a pulse." Like a sunlit field sparkling with life after a storm's gloomy clouds have dissipated, this was the moment of salvation I needed. His tactful prompting encouraged me to take charge.

I felt as if a thousand-pound bag of sand had been lifted from my chest. The elusive knowledge, which moments earlier had been locked away and inaccessible, now resurfaced, the steps flowing into place one by one. A failsafe, my senior resident kept me on track, present in the room to assist as I made decisions and helped navigate the code. I slid the endotracheal tube down the patient's throat, and the respiratory therapist started pushing oxygen into his lungs using a handheld resuscitation bag. As the clinical team performed chest compressions and ventilated the patient—their actions as methodical and meticulous as a ritual—I asked them to pause and shock him. Following protocol, we shocked the patient several times using paddles pressed against his chest, in between aggressively thrusting compressions and administering multiple doses of medications to reclaim the heart back to a viable state.

After several very intense minutes, we were able to regain a normal rhythm and find a pulse. The patient remained unresponsive throughout, with minimal blood pressure. The respiratory therapist connected the breathing tube to the mechanical ventilator. A few more drips were added, and treatment was soon assumed by the attending critical care physician. The crowd withdrew from the room one by one.

The 20-minute experience felt more like hours. I walked out of the room both mentally and physically exhausted, as if I had just run my fastest mile or passed my toughest exam. In reality, it had been my toughest exam.

Since then, I've run hundreds of codes and cared for critically ill patients thousands of times. Despite years of exposure to such emergencies, however, the feeling of palpable anxiety never really goes away.

As with any challenging situation in our daily lives, there's always a mix of randomness and order. In emergencies, this delicate balance becomes exponentially magnified, squeezed into a tiny span of time. The element of uncertainty racks our nerves and muddles our judgment.

I'm lucky to have been born in a time in which attempting to revive a patient doesn't require that I scrub in, don sterile gloves, cut open my patient's chest, and massage the heart directly with my own hands.

When Sherwin Nuland, a third-year medical student at Yale School of Medicine, was faced with a similar situation in the mid-twentieth century, the modern technique I practiced on my patient was not yet available. Dr. Nuland, by contrast, would have surgically opened the patient's chest to massage the heart, performing what was then termed "open-chest compressions" in an effort to maintain a steady flow of blood to the vital organs. This was done for as long as it took to bring an electrical apparatus to the patient's room, that was used to shock the fibrillating heart back into a life-sustaining rhythm. The electrical apparatus at the time—now called an AED (Automatic Electrical Defibrillator)—was a hefty, 200-pound gadget that had to be wheeled from one part of the hospital to another when needed.

If I were to go back in time 70 years to live as a doctor, my outlook toward this medical practice would be markedly different. I would feel the wriggling and squirming heart as I squeezed the malfunctioning organ during resuscitation. In present day, technology allows me to know the rhythm of a heart within seconds by attaching electrodes to a patient's chest and reading the rhythm strip on the ECG monitor. I can instantly connect an AED to a patient's chest and, in a flash, jolt the heart back to its proper rhythm.

. . .

The heart is the composite of billions of cells, each with its own tiny consciousness[1] working to power the master muscle that pumps our bodies with blood. Nature's mystery lies in just how these seemingly simple, tiny entities of energy are able to harmoniously pump fluids through our bodies. It was only in the last century that we came to know so much about the functioning of the heart and what happens when it fails. It took over 300 years of meticulous experiments for us to unravel what provides the horsepower governing this brilliant motion.

Our thinkers and philosophers devoted an enormous amount of

---

[1] Consciousness is used here in the sense that every living cell embodies the property of perceptual awareness that is similar to any other life form. Although a single cell has no independent existence, each cell possesses awareness of its own internal milieu and of surrounding cells through its chemical and hormonal network.

time to attempting to decode nature's secret. Early medieval healers, for instance, explained the movement by way of animal spirits. Another popular theory was that fluids sent from the brain ran through tube-like channels to evoke contractions in the heart.

And then there were mystical theories that portrayed the heart as an emblem of the guardian spirit. Theologians long held reverence for this one organ above all others. Twelfth-century Catholic priest Thomas Aquinas concluded that the heart moves the soul within the human body, and this continuous movement is dictated by the heavens above. The Sacred Heart of Jesus, often depicted as pierced by an arrow, was an object of fervent devotion in Renaissance Italy—representations adorned the walls of churches and temples.

A Renaissance Italian prayer exalted that the heart of Jesus "feels all, knows all, and thinks of all," supporting the notion that it was commonplace in the seventeenth century for people to feel with their hearts. Healers romantically characterized this organ as the origin of human expression, pumping the blood within our bodies in response to our emotions. Powerful feelings would beat our hearts quickly, instantly generating heat. The flame lit inside of lovers, in turn, would gently warm the entire body, invigorating men as it inspired bold acts and awakening women with warmth and tenderness.

Philosophers also believed the heart was capable of independent thought, allowing quixotic ideas to pervade everyday language. Even now, when evoking someone's character, people invariably refer to this part of the body using descriptions like cold, empty, or warm-hearted. The heart occupied a supreme position in the hierarchy of organs because of its spiritual and emotional significance, as well as its physiological importance. It was regarded as the stage upon which the emotional action of a person's life unfolded.

With the arrival of the seventeenth century's Scientific Revolution, much of the fascination around the heart faded. In becoming an emotionless pump at the center of a purely material and mechanical body, it no longer offered a home to thoughts, a nursery to the imagination, or a citadel to the soul.

. . .

In 1775, Danish physician Peter Abildgaard announced that he could use electricity to bring back birds from the dead. Initially trained in medicine, he went on to study veterinary science and conducted many experiments on birds, most notably hens. In one of these experiments, he ran electrical current through the head of a living hen until it fell dead. Abildgaard then applied another electric shock to the head, and to his surprise, the hen made a complete recovery. It "walked around quietly on its feet," and even laid an egg after a few days. While Abildgaard had apparently discovered the principle of cardiac resuscitation, his success was attributed to the mysterious power of electricity and was appreciated as mere curiosity.

By the mid-1700s, the scientific study of electricity was well underway in Western Europe and parts of North America. Benjamin Franklin, a man of many skills—politician, philosopher, and physicist—introduced the idea that all substances were penetrated with what he called "electric fluid." His English counterparts already showed that electricity could be conducted over distances by metal wire.

Electricity's mysterious nature fascinated Franklin. He enjoyed hosting "parties of pleasure" near his Pennsylvania home, to which he'd invite high-profile friends to witness the event's highlight: electrocuting a turkey before turning it into part of the evening meal. Later, his experiments grew more serious. When he failed to kill a large turkey by shocking it, the undeterred Franklin creatively added more "electric bottles" to achieve success. The Royal Society congratulated him on this and similar achievements involving electricity, duly noting them in their proceedings. Before scientists began looking for more constructive uses of electricity, bird-shocking displays were common parlor tricks.

It wasn't until Luigi Galvani (1737–98), a lecturer in anatomy and a professor of obstetrics at the University of Bologna, observed that not only metals but also organic tissue could conduct electricity that the concept of bio-electricity was introduced. Galvani connected the nerves of a freshly deceased frog to a long metal wire and directed it toward the sky during a storm. To his surprise, with each flash of lightning, the dead frog's legs danced as if it had come back to life. This revelation actually went on to become the inspiration behind Mary Shelley's famous *Frankenstein* 20 years after Galvani's death.

Galvani discovered that nerves weren't simply pipes by which bodily fluids traveled—they're electrical conductors. These were the first experiments that ultimately led to the conclusion that life, at the most basic level, is simply a flow of electrons.

But one mystery remained unsolved: Where does this power to excite muscle cells come from?

Alessandro Volta, a popular physicist credited with the invention of the first electric battery, argued in papers published in 1792 that the electric stimulus for the contraction of the muscles came from an outside source. By then, Galvani had already hypothesized that muscle tissue could generate its own electricity—no external source was required. What he was unable to determine was the biochemical underpinning of this mechanism.

Volta became Galvani's intellectual adversary, although there was no personal animosity between the two. The physicist actually built the first battery just to disprove the doctor's theory. This brilliant rivalry led both to complete a number of significant nerve-conduction experiments.

The heart is unlike any other muscle in our body. Weighing merely 10 ounces, a healthy heart beats about 2.5 billion times during the average lifespan of 70 years without any power interruption. Biologists wondered if there must be something particularly special about the electricity generated within this muscle. They theorized it must have unique properties, such as its own spark plug.

Since that time, rather than romanticizing the virtues of the heart or exalting its prowess, we've vigorously experimented on it. We took it apart, piece by piece, testing and retesting it systematically. We discovered that the source of excitation, called the pacemaker, resides within the heart itself. Each pacemaker functions as a battery-powered entity, transmitting signals to different cells to perform uninterrupted excitation. With this understanding, the foundation of a new branch of science—electrophysiology—was born.

. . .

What we now commonly know as CPR—the familiar reaction that leads us to immediately start pounding on an unconscious individual's chest—took nearly a century to perfect. It started when doctors inadvertently sent a young patient into cardiac arrest as the result of a medical misadventure.

During a routine procedure in 1848 in which 15-year-old Hanna Greener was having an infected toe removed, her heart stopped suddenly during the administration of chloroform, a then new and "wondrous blessing" of an anesthetic. It didn't take long for the use of this highly inflammable spirit to backfire on the operating table—Greener, otherwise healthy, was the first victim.

Six years earlier, in 1842, the first surgery using general anesthesia was completed—made possible by ether. Not long after, chloroform rose in popularity as a cheaper, easier anesthetic alternative. Despite its risk of paralysis of vital organs, for many patients, the use of chloroform far outweighed enduring the brutal pain of being awake during an operation.

Until the early 1800s, surgery was akin to torture. Surgeons had to perform amputations and other procedures while the patient remained fully awake. In those days, the skill of a surgeon was measured by how quickly he worked, with slightly less priority given to how well a procedure was executed. The nineteenth-century chemists, however, forever changed how surgery was performed. Humphry Davy, a chemist, was the first to suggest the use of nitrous oxide to alleviate pain.

And surgery wasn't the only situation for which a medicinal use of chloroform proved useful. In 1847, the practice of administering anesthesia to assist with the pain of labor and childbirth was first introduced in England. In 1852, Queen Victoria gave birth to the last two of her nine children with its help and was reportedly delighted.

But not everyone was so thrilled. During the drug's rise, George Bernard Shaw observed, "Chloroform has done a lot of mischief. It's enabled every fool to be a surgeon." A narrow section of clergy were also quick to oppose and protest against these successful attempts to abolish pain, arguing, "Chloroform is a decoy of Satan's, apparently offering itself to bless women, but in the end it will harden society and rob God of the deep, earnest cries which arise in time of trouble for help." The clergy complained that easing labor pains would threaten the foundation of the patriarchal religion, as "the cries of women during childbirth are for the glory of God."

A year after Greener's accidental death, John Snow, the first professional anesthetist, recognized a pattern of chloroform-induced cardiac arrest in its use as a surgical anesthetic. Because no one had discovered yet why the heart went into a standstill, no remedy existed.

As a result, it didn't take long for chloroform to fall out of favor. Ether's staying power as the surgical anesthetic of choice in the mid-1800s can be credited to its wider margin between an effective dose and a toxic one.

Our consideration of sudden death from cardiac arrest evolved dramatically after Dr. John McWilliam diligently experimented with hearts during immediate cardiac standstill. He discovered that, in certain situations, the heart just doesn't stop abruptly; instead, it experiences irregular and uncoordinated contractions known as ventricular fibrillation. Intervening by jolting it back to regular rhythm is called *de*fibrillation.

While working on dogs in 1933, biophysicists proved that directly applying an electrical current and then defibrillating a quivering heart could restore regular rhythm. But the method required first opening the dog's chest, which was obviously a difficult, highly invasive approach. Nevertheless, this was later extended to humans as physicians utilized an open-chest defibrillating approach on patients. After cutting open the sternum, electrodes were placed directly onto a patient's heart to try to jolt it back to a viable rhythm.

No other approach could be as barbaric an attempt to save a person's life. Yet this was the only technique available at the time—at least until the middle of the twentieth century.

. . .

The year was 1947. Claude Beck, an American cardiac surgeon, was involved in the thoracic surgery of a 14-year-old boy who'd suffered from a severe congenital funnel chest. He was healthy in every other sense. During surgery, while Beck was closing up the chest, the boy's heart stopped. Over the course of the next hour, Beck massaged his patient's heart with his gloved hands, followed by direct defibrillation. After two shocks, the trembling heart returned to its regular rhythm.

Three hours post-surgery, the patient's blood pressure returned to normal levels and the child awoke. The boy went on to make a full recovery, with no neurological deficits or other long-term damage whatsoever.

Twenty-five years earlier, Beck had undergone a life-changing experience during his medical training as a surgical intern. A patient was given several inhalations of ether in preparation for surgery. Within seconds, movement of the patient's chest and abdomen were scarcely visible, his face began to turn pale, and his eyes rolled backward. His pulse became imperceptible, and the anesthetist howled, "The patient's heart has stopped!"

Immediately, the surgical resident assisted Beck in carrying out the protocol at the time: calling the fire department and waiting for them to arrive with oxygen-powered respirators in hope of finally resuscitating the patient. Unfortunately, Beck witnessed the death of his patient during this traumatic episode, and he was never the same.

From that day forward, Beck was determined to develop a better way to manage these emergencies—to put the capability of resuscitation into the hands of doctors, not firefighters. He realized that ventricular fibrillation was occurring in hearts that were simply "too good to die," and he set out to do something about it.

He accomplished his first resuscitation using a combination of open-chest cardiac massage and the application of electric current on the exposed heart of a 14-year-old boy in his now famous 1947 surgery.

Despite Beck's success, opening the chest and meticulously placing electrodes directly onto the heart simply took too long. As time is of the essence in all medical emergencies, this procedure was not fast enough for optimal outcomes even in the hands of the most skilled surgeons. It was also limited only to patients who were in the vicinity of a large hospital's surgery suite—meaning that many individuals suffering from cardiac arrest still went untreated.

During cardiac arrest, our whole circulatory system shuts down, cutting off oxygen to vital organs and tissues. Brain cells suffocate and begin to die after only five minutes without oxygen. To prevent irreversible brain damage, the heart has to be returned to normal rhythm as quickly as possible. We needed a better technique, one that didn't involve cutting open a patient's chest every time the heart went into arrest. Though doctors continued to seek an easier method, they came up empty for years. It wasn't a physician but an electrical engineer who finally made the breakthrough we were looking for.

As the popularity of the day-to-day use of electricity grew, so did the number of utility linemen deaths. Soon after, the power company Consolidated Edison of New York selected researchers at Johns Hopkins to study how to reverse the effects of accidental electrocution. William B. Kouwenhoven—described as a pipe-smoking German professor of electrical engineering—joined the research team in 1928.

His first order of business was to develop a method to shock the heart without having to open the chest, which would enable the resuscitation of utility workers in the field. In a surprising discovery, he stumbled across the amazing revelation that counter-shocking the intact chest with electricity could restore the heart to a normal rhythm. Cutting open the chest was no longer necessary. By 1957, the closed-chest defibrillator prototype, a 200-pound box with two insulated cables and copper electrodes, was born.

The concept was simple: When internal electricity fails to excite the heart cells, supply it from the outside. While perfecting the defibrillator, a graduate student on Kouwenhoven's team stumbled upon another game-changing technique. Guy Knickerbocker noticed that even before the current was turned on, when the heavy electrode paddles were pushed against a dog's chest, its blood pressure would rise. Pushing the paddles in the rhythm of a heartbeat—even without electricity—caused circulation to return. This observation meant that with forceful rhythmic pressure applied to the chest, enough blood would flow to sustain vital organs. Ideally, this would give the patient enough time to get to the hospital for further treatment.

The duo was eventually joined by a cardiac surgeon by the name of James Jude. The three spent a year testing their method before publishing a paper on CPR. The results were incredible. The first successful documented case on a human patient involved a 35-year-old woman in 1959. After witnessing the patient go into cardiac arrest, Jude recalled:

> This woman had no blood pressure, no pulse, and ordinarily we would have opened up her chest. Instead, since we weren't in the operating room, we applied external cardiac massage. Her blood pressure and pulse came back at once. We didn't have to open her chest.

Further testing allowed the trio to perfect the details of this new technique—where to press, how fast, how deep. Their findings resulted in another great leap forward in the quest to revitalize hearts that were too good to die.

Thanks to their work, 20 patients at Johns Hopkins received CPR between 1959–1960, and all were resuscitated successfully. Kouwenhoven remarked that "This was the breakthrough we were looking for."

CPR was introduced to physicians in a widespread capacity in 1960. Thanks to how easy it was to train non-medical civilians to perform the technique, it quickly became the forerunner for public use in the event of cardiac arrest. Parents of today's baby boomers were the first generation in history to outwit the age-old conviction that we are powerless against paralysis of circulation.

What made defibrillation such an astounding discovery was that no extensive medical training was needed to perform it. Anyone, anywhere could try to rescue a trembling heart with nothing more than a handheld gadget. Today, the defibrillators that once weighed 200 pounds now weigh just 5, and are available not only in hospitals but in public places like schools, office buildings, and shopping malls throughout the world.

Over time, persistent application of scientific methods helped build public confidence in physicians and re-established trust, making the proverbial bond between doctors and patients stronger than ever before. It made it so strong, in fact, that our perception of death itself changed, owing to the promise of what medicine can offer.

CHAPTER 11

THE UTOPIA OF CURING DEATH

> Life is . . . the totality of functions which resists death.
>
> —XAVIER BICHAT

> Medicine no doubt, has helped us a lot to cure so many diseases, but death still remains an incurable one!
>
> —MEHEK BASSI

On a cold winter morning in 2014, my patient Hazel Steinrich woke up to the morphine wearing off as the pain in her left hip came alive with a piercing stab, a merciless reminder of having gone under the knife the night prior for a full hip replacement. Despite a few hours of sleep, she was overwhelmed with exhaustion—she was tired mostly of lying in bed, an especially difficult circumstance for the peppy, energetic woman accustomed to the vigorous grind of being an ICU nurse.

I'd seen Hazel a day earlier when she was first admitted to the general medical floor. Her orthopedic surgeon wanted me—the attending physician—to clear her for an afternoon surgery. When I'd first entered the room, I noticed Hazel's left leg was clearly turned outward and shorter than the right, indicating she'd sustained a displaced hip fracture. I asked her how she became injured.

"Oh, I'm an idiot," she laughed. "I was in a hurry to get to work this morning, and I slipped on the wet floor in my bathroom and landed on my hip." Her tenor was upbeat as she tried to diminish the true gravity of her injury. I could tell immediately that what bothered her more than the pain was that she was now a patient.

Hazel, who appeared to be in her early sixties, had cared for several of my critically ill patients. During my first days as an attending physician at the hospital, she'd whispered tips on how to field challenging questions from families that I, as a novice, hadn't yet mastered the art of handling.

At her core, Hazel was deeply caring, but she also possessed a shrewd edge—an often-necessary trait in the nursing profession. As she once described it, she didn't "give a crap" for the drama that some patients seemed to crave during their hospital stays. "I've seen enough in my 45 years as a nurse," she told me, defending her pointed attitude.

The truth was, I hadn't ever given much thought to the implications of her timeline—to those "45 years as a nurse." She had a vivacious sense of humor, and even in her most straightforward moments, I found her to be youthfully funny. But when our roles changed and I became her doctor, I was awed to learn that she was some 15 years older than I'd guessed. She'd kept her age well hidden by her tenacious dedication to her work. She seldom showed any signs of defeat from long, toiling shifts.

From her bedside, her daughter Jen whispered tenderly, "We told her many times to be careful. She thinks she's still a spring chicken." This theme of Hazel's supposed youth would come to play a large role in the following months as my patient tried her hardest to outrun her age.

Hazel had sustained a fracture in the top end of her thigh bone, where it snugly fits into the socket of the pelvis; it was snapped in two places and no longer aligned. Generally, in these cases, aged bones will do better if at least some components of the hip are replaced. For Hazel, this meant the replacement of both the ball and the socket—a total hip replacement.

On the day of surgery, just as Hazel had done for so many of her own patients, a nurse changed her into a backless hospital gown, and IVs were started in the backs of both of her hands. She was wheeled to the operation theater, a place all too familiar to her after helping transport hundreds of patients there herself throughout her long nursing career. Her daughter stuck around for as long as she was allowed.

Once Hazel entered the operating room, things moved swiftly. The anesthesiologist started the IV sedative, a cocktail composed of Propofol, Fentanyl, and perhaps Versed. The combo is devised to block pain, wipe out anxiety, and induce amnesia of everything that accompanies the operation. About 90 minutes later, she was greeted by her daughter in the post-operative unit.

The first full day of recovery was rough, which is to be expected after this sort of surgery, especially for someone her age. The next day, a gentle young physical therapist arrived to get Hazel on her feet and test the new joint. Hazel told me that the new hip itself didn't hurt at all, but the suture site sure did. I got the idea that the surgeon and his crew had hyperextended virtually every ligament in her hip while flopping the limb as they chiseled and sawed away, leaving all of her hip muscles more or less sprained.

The usual hospital stay for a total hip replacement is relatively short, and we expected Hazel to be discharged to a rehabilitation facility within a couple of days. Instead, her health took an unexpected turn. Her post-operative course was complicated first by pneumonia and later by kidney failure, as well as a host of treatments in the week that followed.

We worked tirelessly to ensure Hazel's recovery. After an unforeseen and agonizing eight days in the hospital, she couldn't wait to be discharged. She was eventually able to return home after a lengthy stay at a rehabilitation facility, but she was never the same.

Not long after, she retired from nursing. Again and again over the next 10 months, she succumbed to various illnesses, many of which required a hospital visit.

With each attack to her body, she became a little older, a little weaker, and her list of medical problems grew. After receiving the appropriate treatment, she'd perk up within a day or two and appear to have an acceptable quality of life, supported by the caring nursing staff, physical therapists, and physicians who had come to know her so well during her tenure at our hospital.

After every admittance, her entire care team would see her through to recovery and would soon discharge her, optimistic that she'd remain out of the hospital—at least for a while. With a supportive family advocating for her well-being, Hazel had no problems taking her medications and following her dietary and activity recommendations. In theory, she should have been fine.

And sometimes she was. There were times when Hazel would be seen by her primary doctor, who'd evaluate her and conclude she was doing fairly well. But then, a week or so later, she'd be back with new symptoms.

As the number of admissions grew, Hazel's attitude started to change. Her once valiant demeanor was now typified by an uncharacteristic state of dependence. It seemed that she was often relieved to be back in our care because she felt more secure in the company of her medical team. Our familiar faces provided reassurance. Hazel became what's categorized as a hospital-dependent patient.

The frequent hospitalizations and progressive decline in functional status led to a loss of resilience over time. Her body was reaching its physiological limits of recovery. An endless cycle began: Hazel would be discharged, but after no more than a few days, she'd be back again. She suffered from a range of illnesses that included confusion, urinary infections, delirium, contusions from falls, low and high blood sugar and blood pressure, pneumonia, bronchitis, and dehydration. With each hospitalization, the staff would find her health in a worse state than when she'd been discharged a few weeks (or even days) earlier. Eventually, her disappointed and worried family lamented that we must be discharging her too soon, despite the fact that she didn't require an ongoing inpatient stay. To them, their mom was healthy, strong, and able—they'd never seen her in this predicament.

As she weakened, Hazel made more visits to the emergency room, most of which *did* result in lengthier hospital stays. We tried to make her better, and we tried even harder to keep her out of the hospital by transitioning her to temporary rehab facilities. Unfortunately, she often didn't qualify for extended care at these facilities because, at the time of her discharge, she looked "well on chart" to her insurance providers.

The option of a nursing home was discussed, but neither Hazel nor her family felt this was a viable solution. Hazel loved being home with the grandkids and sitting on the front porch—the thought of coaxing her into a nursing home seemed unreasonable to everyone charged with her care.

Hazel's situation wasn't unique. Many elderly patients suffer from multiple chronic conditions and have minimal physical reserve to compensate for the acute stress of an illness. In the 1940s and 1950s, death was more often sudden, the result of a stroke or heart attack. With medical advancements and life-sustaining measures, patients who survive life-threatening illnesses now live longer. Acute decompensations can be corrected with acute-care interventions, such as pacemakers to keep the ticker from slowing down. In many ways, the existence of numerous illnesses, such as chronic heart failure or end-stage kidney disease, is a direct product of the successes and advances of medicine.

Over the next two and a half years, Hazel's health continued to deteriorate. Her heart was losing its resiliency, perhaps from silent heart attacks she'd suffered in months prior. She had no strength or energy left—at times, she didn't even have the energy to breathe in and out on her own. She sunk to the lowest point of her health. She didn't fear death itself, but the suffering from lack of air was an agonizing part of her journey.

Growing weaker and weaker, she decided she preferred to stay at home and die peacefully rather than undergo any more "pointless suffering," as she called it. She made the decision to forgo any further treatment or the medical attention she'd once appreciated while in the hospital. Her family was supportive of her choices, even though their love for her often blinded them to her distress. From time to time her daughter would assert in a pressured tone, "Mom, do you know what will happen if you don't get up and push yourself? You'll die. And we can't let that happen."

Late one evening, I received a call from the emergency department that one of my patients was being admitted to the ICU and was now on a ventilator. That patient was Hazel. I was at a loss of words to learn that she had gone into cardiac arrest at her home.

Jen frantically filled in the emergency line with what had happened: After Hazel had used the restroom earlier that afternoon, she'd become pale and unresponsive, then collapsed. Paramedics arrived in minutes to find her on the ground, pulseless. After two rounds of epinephrine and intubation to provide artificial respirations, the emergency care team was able to resuscitate her. She was rushed to the hospital and placed on a ventilator in the ICU.

The next morning, she was the first patient I rounded. Hazel was nearly unrecognizable—a far cry from the strong, vibrant nurse I'd come to know over the years. Her thin frame was bruised with multiple needle sticks from so many failed attempts to obtain IV access. Because they couldn't find a non-collapsible entry point for an IV, paramedics were required to place an intraosseous needle by drilling into her upper arm bone—a necessity to administer resuscitating and life-sustaining medications directly into the marrow. Her cheeks were distorted from the tape that held the tube down her throat, making her look even less familiar.

It's as though a tube adorned every part of her body—one hung from her nose, another from her neck, a third from her bladder, and two more from either arm, each serving as a painful reminder that she wasn't thriving on her own.

Her sobbing daughter was surrounded by other close members of the family in the waiting room. After I approached to provide an update, Jen ended the conversation with one clear message: Keep her mother alive by "any means necessary."

· · ·

Advances in healthcare over the past century have allowed us to combat many severe illnesses and even delay death, though often at a cost to quality of life. We desire the ability to retain control even in the face of fatal illnesses and at advanced ages. To facilitate this, we've developed many tools as a means of overcoming hurdles to recovery—whatever those obstacles may be.

Cardiopulmonary Resuscitation (CPR) was originally meant to save "hearts that are too good to die," but the promise of technology has also been misleading.

It's interesting to see where we obtain our facts. We like to think that patients learn about CPR from many sources, including physicians, personal accounts from family and friends, and CPR courses. In a number of studies, however, patients report that they obtain much of their information from the media. For example, researchers found that 92 percent of patients over age 62 obtained information about CPR from television and 82 percent from newspapers. In a related study, 70 percent of patients over 74 years old obtained information about CPR from TV.

Patients also tend to overestimate their likelihood of survival after receiving CPR, and this misinformation may lead them to choose to undergo resuscitation in situations in which survival is realistically extremely unlikely.

Rates of long-term survival after cardiac arrest tell a very different story than what's been depicted by our entertainment outlets. In a study of how patients undergoing CPR on television compared with patients in the real world, Dr. Susan Diem and her team at Durham Veterans Affairs Medical Center collected information from the three popular TV shows *ER*, *Chicago Hope*, and *Rescue 911* between 1994 and 1995. On all three shows combined, 75 percent of patients were alive immediately after their cardiac arrests, and 67 percent appeared to survive long term. In reality, the odds of successful recovery from CPR are far more bleak. A reputed study found that only 10 percent of patients in their 40s and 50s successfully recover following the administration of CPR after cardiac arrest. That percentage continues to drop with each decade of life, with a successful resuscitation rate of 8 percent for patients in their 60s and 7 percent for patients in their 70s. Once a patient reaches 80, the chance of successful resuscitation falls to a mere 3 percent.

In another study published in August 2015 by researchers at the University of Southern California, half of the characters who received CPR in two popular television medical dramas (*Grey's Anatomy* and *House*) made enough of a recovery to eventually leave the hospital. In real life, only 13 percent of patients given CPR were found to survive long term.

Through as late as the 1950s, as illnesses robbed us of our grand- or great-grandparents, we would do our best to provide comfort while they had a final chance to share cherished memories with close family in the familiarity of their own homes. Even as their health declined, the elderly continued to do many of the things they enjoyed—chatting with friends, watching the news, reading books, and crocheting blankets for future generations. They passed on while watching their grandchildren play, while saying goodbye to their loved ones, or while sleeping in their own beds.

But almost no one dies at home today. Even though 7 out of 10 of us say we'd prefer to die at home, most of us (more than 70 percent) die in a hospital; a grim passing in intensive care is the common image of modern death. Instead of spending their precious last moments with the ones they love, our elders are surrounded by the noise and energy of strangers, with teams of medical professionals frantically trying to restore a frail body.

Family members, in many instances, are left grappling with their own guilt in the wake of letting go of an ill parent, even when the chances of a meaningful recovery after an intervention are negligible.

Death has been medicalized and orchestrated to such an extent that dealing with it has become alien to almost anyone outside of the medical profession. We became not only incompetent when dealing with the process of dying, but worse. A hypocritical attitude, conventional deception, and artificiality emerge as a dominant motif.

The doctor, disregarding the true feeling of his or her patient, carries on the routine by prescribing more medications and offering more tests—despite being well aware of the inevitable. And the visitors insist on treating him as if he were merely sick instead of dying. The entire act of dying becomes a charade, each party delicately dancing around the truth at hand. The person who is sick can see through the act as visits start to feel more like obligations as opposed to support.

Our adopted attitude to the dying person, this hypocrisy, is perhaps more tormenting than the prospect of mortality itself. In the midst of fears of relinquishing life, the patient yearns for honesty, for a support system built on facing the facts instead of avoiding the truth. Our reluctance to admit this is symptomatic of a larger problem plaguing society as a whole: the inability to acknowledge the unpleasant, yet natural aspects of life and death.

By pushing the limits of the ailing body to extreme measures, we actually perform a strange mockery due to our unwillingness to accept the inevitable passing of the terminally ill person. When someone in that situation says they're sick of the ongoing struggling and incessant medical interventions and would like to simply go, two thoughts often come to our minds. First, we tend to view this coming to terms as a self-destructive act of defiance that connotes a mental illness. Second, we consider ourselves to have failed them—in society's eyes, death has become a strongly repressed event. This is unlike the attitude of our ancestors, who prepared for the passing (and afterlife) of a family member in a celebratory manner, despite the sadness and mourning of the loss.

The ancient and medieval viewpoints of life and death contrast starkly against our current outlook. Today, we take confidence in our assumed ability to control many things that people in ancient times accepted as natural processes of life. Arab and Jewish doctors, for example, asserted that it was unrighteous for physicians to interfere with nature's most powerful lever of control: death. To wish otherwise was to "make oneself impious."

Second-century Roman Emperor Marcus Aurelius wrote in the book, *Meditations*:

> With all meekness and a calm cheerfulness, to expect death as being nothing else but the resolution of those elements, of which every creature is composed. And if the elements themselves suffer nothing by this their perpetual conversion of one into another, that dissolution, and alteration, which is so common unto all, why should it be feared by any? Is not this according to nature? But nothing according to nature can be evil.

In ancient times, death was a transition—we simply perished into something else. A general ease and acceptance surrounded this phase of life. Medieval thought leaders like the Roman statesman Cicero admired how nature conducted human life and progressed us through varying stages. Each stage, like each season, occupied a specific purpose and contained distinguished characteristics. Our fate was nature's will. Old age was seen as a natural phenomenon, not something to try to outrun. Eluding immortality meant distrusting God's final judgment.

The sixteenth and seventeenth centuries brought with them a change to this viewpoint and a growing confidence that we can control nature and therefore hold death at bay.

The radical sixteenth-century German physician Paracelsus argued that if we can preserve a dead body by embalming, we must be able to preserve a living body for an extended length of time. He believed this instinct to control nature with medicine was not blasphemous (as believed by our ancient counterparts), but totally in line with God's plan. According to Paracelsus, God created these medications for our use, so we were at liberty to use them.

Francis Bacon, one of the main drivers of the Scientific Movement, believed that which may be repaired is potentially eternal. He used the analogy of a constantly burning flame in a Roman temple—through ongoing replenishment, it was never allowed to go out. While his idea was relatively straightforward, he knew that prolonging life was easier said than done. "So great a work as the stopping and turning back the powerful course of nature," he observed.

It's astonishing to discover how our perception of death has changed, albeit gradually, from a natural process to something preventable. While this thought was strengthened in the seventeenth century, the seeds for this concept were first sown a few hundred years prior. In the thirteenth century, influential English philosopher Roger Bacon wrote a treatise on longevity, which was published four centuries later in 1683 as *The Cure of Old Age, and Preservation of Youth*.

Chemist Robert Boyle wrote in *Chymical, Medicinal and Chyrugical Adresses* that "within a short time we shall have a universal medicine, which will not only recover the sick and keep them well but also take away death, and forever swallow it up." Boyle, the most famous alchemist of his time, spent most of his life experimenting to discover the promise of immortality.

Benjamin Franklin, the eighteenth-century inventor and revolutionary diplomat, famously joked that nothing in life is certain except death and taxes. He, too, was enthralled by the possible prolongation of life. "It is impossible to imagine the height to which we may be carried, in a thousand years, the power of man over matter," he once wrote, regretting that he was "born too soon." Like his predecessors, he had faith that eventually we'd conquer old age and lengthen our lives "at pleasure."

As time marched on, so too did the expectations on medical science and its troopers, the physicians. In *The Martyrdom of Man*, written in 1872, Winwood Reade predicted that "disease will be extirpated; the causes of decay will be removed; immortality will be invented." And expectations have grown even higher as the twenty-first-century project is now to view death itself as a terminal illness, where aging is its risk factor. In general, we define risk factors as that which can be prevented before damage has occurred—90 percent of lung cancers are due to cigarette smoking, for instance, and quitting lowers the risk. The idea of casting aging as a risk factor for the terminal condition called death intoxicates researchers in the field who pride themselves on the ability to push the limits of evolution.

. . .

Our perception of death has changed with time as we've attempted to outrun mortality through advances in medicine. The major medical triumph—longer life expectancy—is the result of three main factors: a reduced infant-mortality rate; prevention of communicable diseases; and the prolongation of old age by tackling acute illnesses such as strokes, heart attacks, and kidney failure. Yet this third factor comes at a price.

Motorized wheelchairs and portable oxygen tanks have become

emblems of rising age. Liberal use of medical interventions such as heart bypass surgeries and kidney dialysis is already routine (and becoming more common with time) at the oldest of ages. This exemplifies the successes of life extension, as well as the burden this success places on family members and society as a whole.

We as a society were not prepared to deal with the challenges brought forth by prolonging life. Despite world wars, genocides, and pandemics, the life expectancy in many parts of the world over the past two centuries has risen by about three months per year. This is true even without the full potential of biotechnology available to the masses. The rate of increased life expectancy may soon accelerate rapidly as genetics and biotech advance.

We're at a phase in scientific evolution in which we're able to prevent many causes of sudden death, but we're still struggling to deal with declining quality of life at old age. If we reduce the risk of heart disease, we live long enough to succumb to cancer. If we win over cancer, Alzheimer's robs us of our quality of life. Meanwhile, our immune system wears out just as our bones do, putting us at increased risk of infections, falls, fractures, and almost every other common condition. Technological innovation is betting on replaceable human parts and genetic bioengineering, even reverse aging, but we are far from that.

Over the past century, we've done a magnificent job of converting fatal diseases into chronic conditions. Heart attack survivors may end up with congestive heart failure, patients with acute kidney disease may have to live with end-stage kidney failure, and stroke survivors may have to endure long-term debility with feeding tubes and bed sores.

This idea that we could hypothetically elongate the terms of all phases of life has led to a disappointing realization. While we could increase our lifespans, we haven't yet discovered a way to prolong youth. What we've accomplished instead is the less preferred alternative: We've extended old age. By systematically turning certain killer diseases into chronic conditions, we've undesirably prolonged the final third of our lives.

It is a well-known phenomenon that evolutionary forces favor the young by providing them with strength and verve. This is exemplified in the wild, where young animals always far outnumber the old. But we've defied this evolutionary principle, and today, we live in a society where the elders far outnumber the young—a trend that is only expected to continue. It's estimated that, on a global level, the 85-and-over population is projected to increase 350 percent between 2010 and 2050.

Many qualities that are favorable during our youth become disadvantageous as we age, typified by a decrease in vitality and an increase in vulnerability. Estrogen, for instance, allows a young woman to bear offspring, but as we've implemented replacement treatments for older women, the result can mean a higher risk for ovarian cancer. A high testosterone level in young age gives men strength and vigor, whereas it makes them more susceptible to prostate cancer in later stages of life. It has never been in evolution's best interest to expand life expectancies beyond a certain point, simply for the fact that resources need to be freed up for the young. In this sense, aging and death can be regarded as an evolved adaptation of species. As Warthin (1929) observed:

> We live but to create a new machine of a little later model than our own, a new life-machine that in some ineffable way can help along the great process of evolution of the species somehow more efficiently than we could do were we immortal. The Universe, by its very nature, demands mortality for the individual if the life of the species is to attain immortality.

The only evolutionary mechanism that rewards longevity is when the social group draws adaptive benefits from the existence of older generations that play a greater role in the success of their grandchildren.

It's beneficial when older individuals are regarded as repositories of knowledge, imparters of valuable information, and mediators of social tensions. But as we've phased out of tribe living and shifted more toward a self-sufficient smaller family unit—from collectivism to individualism— even the small trace of evolutionary favorability of senility is becoming lost.

Contrary to the notion that worn-out tissue cannot renew itself, we've invented ways to outsmart nature because we've become convinced that it's worth the effort. It's human nature that unless we totally believe in something, we won't be able to put our hearts and minds to it. The concept of death is no different, and many experts have poured all their efforts into the task of preventing it. Because we've taken up this project of extending life so enthusiastically, we've been able to discover many ways to prolong it.

Eastern civilizations, however, maintain a perception of mortality that's changed much less over thousands of years. People in many Asian cultures continue to believe in the circular notion of life, viewing birth and death as a looped continuum. The premise is based on rebirth, in which death of one life is continued as the rebirth of something new.

But for many of us, as the children of the free-thinking scientific era, there's no such thing as our "next life." Instead, life is unidirectional and finite, and because of this we've tacitly determined to prolong the lifespan of *this* organism. The result, oftentimes, is a sorrowful lengthening of our worst years.

But utopia looms. "Eventually, the process of aging, which is unlikely to be simple, should be understandable. In fact, in the next century, we shall have to tackle the question of the preferred form of death," Francis Crick asserts in *The Humanist* in 1986.

Doctors take great pride in eradicating diseases. Physicians don't like to give up on people, and many patients like it when their doctors refuse to do this as well. As the German doctor Christoph Hufeland observed in *The Art of Prolonging the Life of Man* in 1797, "Long life is as at all times the chief wish, and the principal object of mankind." The unrelenting project of medical science is ultimately the immortality of human flesh.

As my patient Hazel's health continued to deteriorate with no meaningful recovery, a wave of resolve rushed over her family as they realized almost in unison that it was time to stop prolonging the inevitable—it was time to put their mother's comfort first. They withdrew aggressive measures in order to ease her exit from the world. After only a couple hours, surrounded by her loving family, Hazel passed away. Her peace led to retrospective regret on the part of her surviving children—why had they waited so long and fought so hard just so their mom could suffer for a few more months? "We thought she would pull off a miracle," they reasoned.

CHAPTER 12

HOW DOCTORS LOST THE NARRATIVE

> In examining disease, we gain wisdom about anatomy and physiology and biology. In examining the person with disease, we gain wisdom about life.
>
> —OLIVER SACKS

> *Taceant colloquia. Effugiat risus. Hic locus est ubi mors gaudet succurrere vitae.*
> Let conversation cease, let laughter flee.
> This is the place where death delights to help the living.
>
> —GIOVANNI MORGAGNI, EIGHTEENTH-CENTURY ANATOMIST

With a heart functioning at only 30 percent, 63-year-old Maria Frances was admitted to the hospital where I worked with congestive heart failure and chronic obstructive pulmonary disease (COPD). Her health was deteriorating, and she was close to depending on an oxygen tank 24/7 in order to breathe.

Her three adult children sat by her side, concerned but frustrated. When I asked Maria about her latest symptoms, her son, a 35-year-old paramedic, sighed. "It's her drinking." Maria's heart doctor had diagnosed her recently with alcoholic cardiomyopathy—heart failure due to long-term alcohol abuse.

"And we asked her to quit smoking, but it doesn't matter—she does it anyway," her eldest daughter added, looking away as she spoke, clearly exhausted from years of not being heard.

The reality, though, is that sometimes we choose to participate in unhealthy behaviors even when we're aware of the consequences, or despite wanting to stop. I kept a neutral tone when I asked Maria why she continued to drink and smoke.

"I'm stressed at work," she answered, "so I'll come home and drink a few beers. Three, four maybe. I'll have a few cigarettes throughout the evening, then try to get some sleep." She seemed slightly embarrassed to reveal her vices. Behind her, Maria's daughter rolled her eyes and signaled to me that this was just the tip of the iceberg, and the other two children nodded in agreement. Their mother's drinking, they suggested, was far worse than she was letting on.

Maria continued, "I hardly get much sleep." She worked as the manager of a department store, and she cited increasing demands at her job as the primary instigator of her unhealthy lifestyle choices. Even though her children resided nearby, she lived alone.

I suspected there was more to the story. No matter what treatment options we were able to offer, until we could uncover what was driving Maria's choices, her physical health would continue to spiral.

The next day during my visit, Maria was alone, without the pressure of her children listening in. Her breathing was better, and she was hopeful that a release from the hospital was within reach and she could get back to her routines.

I asked her the same question from the previous day, but in a slightly different tone: "Tell me why the drinking and smoking?" This time, her response unfolded a bigger picture, putting her habits and health into perspective.

When Maria was 23, she had given birth to her first child. Around that same time, her husband experienced a ruptured brain aneurysm, requiring major surgery. Young, scared, and overwhelmed, Maria turned to the occasional drink to cope. Two years later, smoking entered the picture, and two children followed soon after. Eventually, as a result of his ill health, her husband was no longer able to financially provide for the family, leaving Maria as the sole earner and caregiver for her husband and kids. Despite many attempts to quit, Maria's unrelenting dependence on these unhealthy habits only grew stronger. Years of alcohol abuse took a toll on her heart as the smoking destroyed her lungs.

Maria spoke highly of her family, blaming only herself for the choices she'd made over the years concerning her health. Ultimately, she shared her regret that alcohol and smoking had become such a major part of not only her life, but of the lives of her beloved children. She was thankful, at least, that her children learned from witnessing her dependency and failing health not to follow in her footsteps.

Maria's grief and regret were palpable as she poured out her heart to me. "They mostly stay away from me now because of my habits. They don't want their children around a bad influence," she said, wiping away her tears.

When her children arrived for their next visit, I narrated the story back to them: Raising three children all by herself and struggling to thrive in both motherhood and the workplace for so many years without a break had resulted in an ultimate breakdown of Maria's health. It was a case of fragile lungs and a failing heart within a worn-out body. The drinking and smoking had contributed to her poor health, yes, but they were also a symptom of an even bigger health issue—the years of stress and pressure Maria had endured as she took care of her family.

A sense of guilt dawned, and now the children seemed more apologetic than annoyed. Although they'd always been aware of their mother's struggles, for years they were unable to see beyond the idea that Maria was nothing more than "a weak addict" who "did this to herself." But after hearing her familiar story from a medical professional, they seemed to understand her predicament with a renewed outlook: She was a tenacious woman put in an unthinkably challenging situation, and she did her best to keep going for the sake of her family. They remained silent, listening intently with tears in their eyes as they held their mother's hands.

Without a complete narrative, we had been unable to provide Maria with care that was the most useful to her. We could have, for the tenth or twentieth time, recommended that Maria cut back on the drinking and smoking or try to get more sleep. But in this case, helping to identify the underlying cause of Maria's behavior was a critical step toward her recovery. She needed a stronger and more active support system in the form of her children, and she needed to take realistic steps to practice better and more consistent self-care.

The story behind Maria's illness provided a framework for approaching her problems holistically, addressing both her physical and mental well-being. Had I just addressed her heart and lungs, she'd continue to self-medicate her emotional problems. And as she remained set in those habits, her children would continue to distance themselves from her, perpetuating the cycle.

Patient narratives like these give us a window into why it matters to address deeply emotional qualities such as hurt, despair, anger, hope, grief, and moral conflict. These feelings frequently accompany, and may even contribute to, a patient's illness. This is the art of medicine in its best form.

However, like many of my colleagues, the reality is that I underinvest in vivid, narrative-based engagement with many of my patients. I typically don't start my patient interviews with "Tell me your story." Doctors rarely have the time to sit and listen while the tales of their patients unfold. In fact, though we try to mine for clues from the brief exchanges in which we engage, the relentless avoidance of such encounters with patients is not uncommon in medical practice. James Tulsky, chair of the Department of Psychosocial Oncology and Palliative Care at the Dana-Farber Cancer Institute in Boston, conducted a series of studies showing that senior oncologists responded appropriately to patient expressions of negative emotion only slightly more than one in five times. Some physicians worry that discussing such emotions would lead them down a rabbit hole and consume huge amounts of their already limited time.

Sure, the financial demands of our current medical practice necessitate speed and shortcuts. While the common reason for such emotional distance is that doctors are pressured to mind the clock while they examine patients, there's actually an even more organic reason for avoidance of patients' personal stories.

Imagine the typical day of an oncologist. She sees 20 patients in her office, and every one of them is going through an existential crisis. They're either anxious to hear the result of that biopsy report after a trial of chemo or to learn the result of a follow-up CT scan after the completion of radiation treatment. The oncologist has to get through each day without becoming emotionally exhausted herself.

In the midst of loaded existential situations during which decisions can have a life-altering impact on a patient, there can be enormous emotional distress not just for the families, but for the physician, too. This is not a modern phenomenon—it's human nature, a survival mechanism to protect oneself from succumbing to the negative emotions of others.

Emotions exploit our intellectual thinking. When most of us see someone deeply distressed, our own mental responses are triggered—we literally share the suffering of the person we're observing or with whom we're interacting. When we witness a fellow human being in physical pain or anguish, the pain centers in our own brains are activated as if we were experiencing the pain ourselves. Research indicates that for many of us, the effects of emotional contagion apply even when we observe a stranger suffering from distress. This is because our brains cannot clearly distinguish between what we feel and what others feel.

The result: Observing a person in a stressful situation can also induce our own bodies to produce more stress hormones. Evolutionary biologists say that being affected by someone else's emotional state was the earliest step in our evolution as a collaborative species. Empathy served as a bonding mechanism for mutually beneficial cooperation.

It's important for doctors to resist the urge to succumb to patients' feelings. In many critical situations, physicians are far more effective when they're able to maintain a level of detachment and objectivity. It's imperative for physicians to provide care to ailing patients compassionately and to listen without being leveled by the emotions of those under their watch. Now the tough job is to train physicians to be both empathetic and detached at the same time.

. . .

The first time I witnessed the act of death up close was in the earliest days of my clinical rotations. I was a third-year medical student, ill-prepared despite how much I'd attempted to convince myself otherwise. My eyes were fixed on Sarala, a 36-year-old with severe asthma, as she panted until she had no breaths left, and until only that terrible silence remained. Her eyelids were locked in partial closure. Her jaw fell slightly open, instantly becoming prominent and stiff as her face turned pale, cold. I couldn't look away, nor could I endure looking at her.

Seeing someone die incapacitates us. It shows no mercy. The death rattle is hard to erase from memory, and the visual image of the hapless woman remains in the depths of my mind, even now, some 20 years later.

Her teenage son, confused and frightened, was at her bedside while we tried everything in our power to resuscitate her.

Those were the days of my medical training in India, when ventilators were limited and the care of critically ill patients was suboptimal, certainly not up to par with Western standards. After the incident, we found ourselves consoling our sobbing colleague while the senior resident supervising us busied himself with evening rounds, seemingly unshaken with what had just occurred. For him, it was just another day in the hospital ward.

Sometimes it would be best if we could simply erase certain memories, but of course it doesn't work that way. Perhaps some things are meant to be remembered. As a doctor in the making, maybe for me this was a key part of the desensitization I needed to become a better practitioner. To be a physician, my ability to mitigate my emotions while handling a situation was essential so that I could think rationally and objectively, at least until I'd made it to the other side of a critical moment. Perhaps this was a necessary step toward developing that skill. After a few such experiences, dying patients didn't instill in me the same emotional reaction. By degrees, it has since become easier to look away.

I remember my earliest days as a medical student. Cutting through the toughened skin of cadavers with my fellow rookie classmates, we would sometimes ponder, *This could have been me or someone I love.* For many of us, it was the most emotionally grueling task we'd performed to date. As we walked in for the exercise, there was a precipitous silence that felt even more daunting than the row of bodies wrapped in formaldehyde-soaked sheets. Formalin stung our eyes, the smell repugnant. Some of us wanted to walk right back out, but we endured.

As students, we knew almost nothing about the individuals whose bodies we were about to dissect except for their age and sometimes how they'd died. We'd wonder about the life and backstory of the person while observing a missing kidney or an artificial heart valve. We'd sometimes make assumptions based on an arm tattoo or bright red fingernail polish on a frail, wrinkled body—*Was this once a playful woman with a story to tell?* A rare and startling discovery of a five-month-old fetus we once found in a woman as we dissected her uterus became nearly impossible to erase from our young minds; most of us were only about 18 or 19 when we began our training.

For the first time in our lives, we were expected to shift our focus from the awe and angst evoked by death and nudity to the intellectual exercise of learning. We could have done this a little later in our training, but instead we began the very first day—a perfect initiation into the profession. The eighteenth-century surgeon William Hunter befittingly remarked that dissecting corpses gave students "necessary inhumanity." It's part of what helped us develop the essential callousness that would protect us from yielding to the distress of tormented patients that was to come. As first-year medical students, we were frequently taunted by the seniors: "You're going to see much worse than this."

We were expected to cut through the bodies with the sharpest knives we'd ever handled. The surgeon's knife was so sharp that if it sliced you, you might not even realize right away that you'd been cut. And even though I knew there was no feeling left in the cadavers, a part of me worried about inflicting pain to the bodies as I cut through the dead skin. It took a conscious effort not to feel like I was hurting them somehow. Within just days, though, I was able to detach myself from the emotional side of the exercise as I, along with the four other students in my group, methodically followed our instructions.

Like a mechanic who takes apart the various components of a car, we started laying open the cadaver and removing the insides tissue by tissue—studying the details of the subcutaneous fat, muscle layers, ligaments, tendons, nerves, and blood vessels with utmost attention until we reached the core: the bones. Moving down from the shoulder, we'd disarticulate one joint at a time until nothing was left. With each training session, we went through rituals of dehumanization as we stepped closer and closer toward mastering the human anatomy.

Our frantically firing neurons and high-geared emotions quieted as we learned to focus on the technical side of dissection. The words of eighteenth-century physician Giovanni Morgagni, "This is the place where death delights to help the living," were called to mind once we started seeing corpses as educational tools. Thus began a new chapter in our lives, the rite of passage into a world where constant exposure to disease and death was the norm.

. . .

The celebrated twentieth-century clinician and teacher Sir William Osler—best known for saying, "Listen to your patient, he is telling you the diagnosis"—argued in his 1912 essay "Aequanimitas" that by neutralizing their emotions to the point that they felt nothing in response to suffering, physicians could "see into" and hence "study" the patient's "inner life."

But this doesn't come easily. In fact, there's an abundance of emotional reactions in first-year medical students as they tend to relate more to patients. In the autumn of 1600, an English medical student studying with the young William Harvey remarked of Italy's San Francesco patients, "These wretched creatures are the most miserable and deplorable objects to exercise upon, both men and women, young and old." In return, Harvey replied, "I observed terrible things with much nausea and loathing," adding that he had tried but failed to forget them. The noxious smells especially disturbed him as he struggled to overcome his rookie queasiness.

Like mirrors, medical students reflect the patient's every sentiment. By the time these students receive their medical degrees, however, these mirrors no longer exude the same level of empathy they once did. In fact, research suggests that with training, physicians' empathy wanes by the third year of medical school, right as students shift from academics to clinical care.

Being that empathy is such an inherent human tendency, scientists became curious as to what it looks like in a physician's brain. A study led by Jean Decety, professor of psychology and psychiatry at the University of Chicago, offered some insight. Decety placed scalp electrodes on physician and non-physician control subjects and had both groups look at images of people either being pricked by a needle or touched with a cotton swab. The electrodes recorded Event Related Potentials (ERPs), which are electrical shifts in brain responses linked to specific stimuli. Whenever non-physicians saw someone in pain, their ERP recordings showed heightened spurts of brain activity, a reaction associated with conscious recognition of what the person in the picture was experiencing.

Interestingly, doctors didn't seem to show any difference in activity regardless of whether they saw people with the cotton swab or the needle—neither image evoked ERPs. What this suggests is that physicians' training teaches their brains to down-regulate the negative arousal most people feel when they witness another's pain.

Tactfully built into physicians' training is the ability for them to move from *feeling more, thinking less* to *feeling less, thinking more.* Over time, we begin to think of a patient's symptoms—such as pain, distress, or bleeding—in biological terms rather than in emotional ones. This exercise also guards against the personal distress, burnout, and compassion fatigue that can result from constant exposure to traumatic visuals.

John Abernathy was a shrewd eighteenth-century surgeon who could tie off a bleeding carotid artery in the neck or a ruptured aneurysm of the iliac artery inside the abdomen when no other surgeon dared. But he had a weakness: He almost never managed to complete a surgery without vomiting. Once he was found by his assistant in the retiring room after an operation with big tears in his eyes, "lamenting the possible failure of what he had just been compelled to do by dire necessity."

Surgeons find detachment to be a necessity in the operating room. But when the circumstance is different—for instance, if the surgeon is letting a patient know that she found metastatic cancer—she still needs to be able to engage her patient with a certain degree of empathy. This, however, contrasts markedly with the ordinary meaning of empathy as feeling into or being moved by another's suffering.

When it comes to the medical profession, what a physician experiences is not empathy in its truest sense. A better description would be "detached concern" or "passionate detachment." Due to the verbosity of such terms, however, twentieth-century medical literature hesitantly settled on calling it "empathy."

The concept of empathy was first discussed in 1873 by Robert Vischer, a German art historian and philosopher who used the word *Einfuhlung* to address a person's emotional reaction to art. Contrary to today's usage, the German term was originally used not to describe an interpersonal attribute, but only to portray the individual's feelings when appreciating beauty.

In 1897, the German psychologist-philosopher Theodor Lipps borrowed the word *Einfuhlung* from aesthetics and applied it to psychology. In describing the personal experiences associated with the concept of *Einfuhlung*, Lipps indicated that he felt an emotional resonance—being moved by another's experience.

The usual meaning of empathy was redefined again when it came to doctors. The medical profession interprets empathy as the act of acknowledging the emotional state of another without experiencing that state oneself. To balance the act of feeling and thinking, medical education implicitly trains doctors to function at two levels at the same time—to be involved and detached simultaneously.

As medical science rapidly advances to discover more diseases and more mechanisms to treat them, the balance consequently shifts to exclusive thinking and imperceptible feeling. After all, the goal of all medical advancements is ultimately to focus solely on the patient's illness with an eye on the cure (whereas nurses' training aims more at caring for the whole individual).

Technical proficiency is vital to any doctor, but his or her expertise can't get in the way of the ability to connect with a patient. In reality, however, it usually does. As a result, when it comes to physicians, compassion becomes predominantly a cognitive exercise, contrasted with a highly emotional response. This mindset is reflected even in a physician's attire. Despite its connotation of serenity, the doctor's white coat, being devoid of color, also represents an emotional neutrality.

One undue consequence of such a highly cerebral exercise becomes quite obvious when doctors encounter terminally ill patients. Instead of engaging in the emotional distress of a patient, perhaps by saying, "You look terrified. Tell me about it," the physician immediately breaks into questions like "How's your pain today? On a scale of 1–10, what would you rate it? How's your nausea? How's the chemo going?"

Physicians lose the much-valued narrative competence to recognize, absorb, metabolize, interpret, and provide sympathetic feedback to the sick because they strive hard not to be moved by the stories of illness.

I once had a patient with severe emphysema. Despite our best efforts, all treatments failed. His lungs were so frail that we were not able to wean him off of ventilator support. The 72-year-old man's wife was very involved in his care right from the beginning. It came time for her to make the tough decision of switching from aggressive treatment to providing comfort measures only. We stepped into the hall and she told me, "I completely understand intellectually," saying this, she pointed to her head, "that he's dying, and I don't see any options but to simply keep him comfortable at this point. But emotionally," now she pointed to her heart, "I just can't convince myself to make this decision." Intellectual understanding of an illness and our emotional reaction to it can be two parallel tracts impossible to converge. Doctors, in such situations, have a responsibility to help patients and their families bridge this difficult divide.

Often, doctors find themselves at a loss for words when a patient asks, "Am I going to die?" or, "Do you think I have only a few more months to live?" I get asked these questions regularly from some of the hospitalized patients I treat. Like my peers, my response typically veers toward a rundown of mortality statistics, and I'm usually single-mindedly focused on curing the disease. In many ways, the thought of a patient dying elicits a connotation of failure.

For doctors, caring and comforting the dying is, at best, a negligible part of our training because the principal goal of medicine is to cure. Dying is a messy business. When training modules on death and dying are covered as part of medical schooling, this information predominantly comes by way of lecture, with student education usually kept restricted to classrooms.

The inclination of doctors to resign from caring for dying patients dates back to a time period that roughly corresponds to the beginning of the Scientific Revolution in Western Europe (although there is probably no causal relation between the two events). When the Hippocratic *corpus* containing the code of ethics for physicians was translated into Latin in 1525, some of the precepts were modified. Despite the diminishing role of Hippocrates and his teachings, some physicians took advantage of his fame to promote their own agendas within the profession. This sixteenth-century version of the medical texts openly advised doctors who wanted "glory" to be careful in choosing their patients. In fact, the texts were changed to reinforce the message that the ethical behavior of doctors is even said to include such glory. They explicitly advised the doctor to avoid a "bad one" by refusing to take on a case where the patient was clearly going to die.

The possibility of a cure is what fuels the collective consciousness of the medical community, and this thinking became emblematic of the modern physician. The direct consequence of such an approach is that doctors tend to resign at the juncture of terminal illness in a patient, concluding that their role as a healer ends the moment there is no longer prospect for a cure.

Patients with incurable illnesses deserve to have their physical, emotional, and existential needs better met, yet preparation for this level of service is largely left out of doctors' training in most medical schools. One significant step forward in improving this necessary and inclusive treatment for terminally ill patients came from someone with a nursing background. Cicely Saunders completed nursing school at St. Thomas' Hospital Nightingale School of Nursing in 1944, a little over 100 years after Nightingale founded her now-famous nursing program. After working for a few years as a nurse and then as a social worker, Saunders grew increasingly distressed by how inadequately the total needs of dying patients were being addressed. She determined that these care methods required reassessment to better treat patients who knew death was near.

"It's the doctors who desert the dying, and there's so much to be learned about pain. If you don't do it properly you'll only be frustrated, and they won't listen to you," said surgeon Norman Barrett in an effort to encourage Saunders to become a doctor so she would be further empowered to alleviate her patients' suffering. At age 33, she returned to St. Thomas' Hospital, this time to enroll in medical school. Shortly after Saunders's acceptance, she wrote an article outlining her ideas regarding a new approach to the end of life:

It appears that many patients feel deserted by their doctors at the end. Ideally the doctor should remain the center of a team who work together to relieve where they cannot heal, to keep the patient's own struggle within his compass, and to bring hope and consolation to the end.

Even as a physician, Saunders's driving force wasn't her medical degree but the emotional needs of her patients and their families. As a result, she founded the hospice movement in 1967. She sought to address "total pain" and thus alleviate the seemingly "pointless" suffering of her terminally ill patients. Total pain was inclusive of physical, emotional, social, and spiritual distress—all of which she faithfully tried to ease through the efforts of hospice. While she was developing this care model, a few moral and philosophical questions arose: How could she ensure that hospice wasn't viewed simply as a death house? How would the traditions of religious charities be interpreted in an increasingly secular world? Lastly, how could it support a staff who had to provide the utmost compassionate care that reached the deepest levels of suffering?

Hospice philosophy was built broadly on the existential needs of the sick—with no pressure on anyone, staff or patient, to participate in religious worship. It was Saunders's roots in nursing and social work that gave her the capacity to think so compassionately about patient care at terminal stages and establish the practice. In 2005, Sanders died of cancer at the age of 87 at the very hospice she first founded.

Since the introduction of hospice in the United States in the 1970s, millions of patients have been assisted. An estimated 1.6 million individuals received hospice care in 2014 alone, and millions more around the world are currently in need of such care.

While Saunders didn't invent a new method of caring for the terminally ill, she did return a much-needed lost wisdom to the healing profession—a wisdom that many modern doctors would benefit from incorporating into their practice today.

PART FIVE

NECESSARY
COMPROMISES

"As we dig deeper into the mysteries of our own biology, we're faced with a counterintuitive phenomenon that our ancient and medieval healers could never have conceptualized: The more experience a physician accumulates, the more out-of-date some aspects of his or her practice are likely to become."

CHAPTER 13

PRICE TAGS

> We may have great and imposing buildings, the last word in hygienic and sanitary appliances, dazzling operation rooms and laboratories, but that stricken human being lying there has many needs that none of these can satisfy.
>
> —MARY NUTTING, A PIONEER IN NURSING EDUCATION,
> IN A TALK TO A GROUP OF COLLEGE WOMEN
> ENTERING NURSING TRAINING IN 1918

The year was 1875. The Royal Charter was bestowed on Belford Hospital in England. In October, a newspaper article announced the new building for the nurses' training school. The announcement read:

Who so powerful a fellow laborer with the wise physician? Who so efficient an assistant to the skillful surgeon as a loving, tender, neat-handed, trained nurse? She is as necessary for the cure of disease as the doctor; nay the recovery from illness depends almost more upon the careful watchful nurse than the prescriptions of the physicians. He sees the patient for a few minutes, she watches hour by hour through the long watches of the silver night.

Until the late 1800s, the nursing profession was quite different from what we see today, although the role was conceptually similar. Nursing duties involved preparation of both the patients' and their own food, washing the ward floors, and attending to the needs of patients who were confined to bed. Staff nurses had long hours and mostly resided in hospitals.

For this reason, nursing was seen as more of a calling than a profession. The tradition dominated the care of the sick during the pre-medieval period, when benevolent outreach of churches and temples included feeding the hungry; caring for the poor; and offering hospitality to widows, children, and strangers—in addition to nursing the ill. The arrangement was originally called "hospitium," the Latin root for *hospital* that is also related to *hospitality*. This religious culture of charity continued with the rapid outgrowth of monastic orders in the fifth and sixth centuries and extended into the Middle Ages.

Monasteries added wards, where caring was meant to provide comfort and spiritual sustenance. Religious orders predominated in medieval nursing, in both Western and Eastern institutions. In the medieval period in the West, for instance, Benedicts ordered that "for these sick brethren let there be assigned a special room and an attendant who is God-fearing, diligent, and solicitous."

One of the most important functions of these monastery wards was the preparation for death—a way to provide for those who failed to recover. Nuns and monks remained with dying individuals throughout the day and night, praying and reading from the scriptures by candlelight. This vigil ensured a "proper passing" by honoring life based on the firm belief that no one should be left to die alone.

These monastic hospitals were also called infirmaries (which literally meant *a sick house*) and were run by nuns and monks who were typically selected for the job due to their diligence, solitude, and practical healing techniques. Medicinal knowledge was acquired informally through experience, as well as through the consultation of manuscripts available in the monastery's library. At the time, there were no formal institutions to train nursing staff.

Guest houses were also turned into wards to care for travelers and the poor. In the early medieval period, though, these guest houses were difficult to come by, due in large part to the lack of nursing staff willing to provide care outside of monasteries. The wealthy, conversely, were often tended to in their own residences.

Eventually, out of necessity, hospitals were built. The growing number of hospitals were financed by local rich aristocrats as a service to the poor immediately following the outbreak of the Black Death in 1348. By this time, Western Europe saw the birth of large universities in France and Italy where physicians could train. In contrast to monastic institutions, these newly built hospitals employed university-educated medical practitioners.

Initially, however, hospitals were frequently attached to monasteries and other places of worship, preserving both the symbolic and material link to religion. Based on the long-established belief that the body and the soul were mutually connected, physicians often refused to treat patients who had not made a confession, as it was thought the sacrament of confession purified the soul from sins. In this way, hospitals continued to emulate monasteries for many years.

· · ·

The rise of the modern hospital began in Paris during the French Revolution. At this time, the scientific approach helped the practice of medicine grow more streamlined, and large-scale innovations within the field added complexity to the profession. Bigger hospitals blossomed throughout Europe, helping to facilitate medical training based on experimental sciences. At last, the humoral holistic model of healing was transformed to the disease-oriented paradigm we know today.

When the cure of the body and care of the soul were separated, many hospitals became more secular. Several maintained some level of religious affiliation, though the sole priority of most hospitals has been to serve the medical needs of patients. These facilities evolved into places where the sick would go for recovery and cure that were based on scientific research rather than faith.

Even as medical treatment was becoming more scientific, the duties of nurses remained more or less the same and still included a great deal of housekeeping and administrative work. This involved the care and management of kitchens, linen rooms, drug rooms, and other supply departments, as well as actual cooking, scrubbing, and laundry. Training for nurses, in tandem with scientific advances, was grossly lacking.

It wasn't until the founding of the modern nursing profession by Florence Nightingale in the mid-1800s that new standards of training were established.

Born in Italy to a rich landlord, Nightingale was a clever and rebellious young woman who never felt at home in the aristocratic circles within which her family moved. Nursing was considered a trade beneath women in the upper classes, and Nightingale bucked tradition by pioneering the profession as we know it during 1854's Crimean War. When she was tapped by England's Secretary of War Sidney Herbert to organize a corps of nurses to tend to Crimea's soldiers, Nightingale put together her team and set sail for the Russian peninsula within days. When the three dozen nurses arrived at Scutari, the British base hospital in Constantinople, they found the conditions even more horrifying than what they'd been warned about. Infectious diseases like typhoid and cholera were rampant, responsible for killing more soldiers than the battle itself.

Nightingale wasted no time. She ministered patients herself at all hours of the day and night. Carrying a lamp through the darkened hallways after sundown, she was nicknamed "the Lady with the Lamp" and "the Angel of the Crimea." The sincerity of her compassionate effort reduced the death rate at the hospital by two-thirds during the year and a half she was there.

But her time in Crimea took its toll. During her tenure at Scutari, Nightingale herself contracted Crimean Fever, an illness from which she never fully recovered. She was bedridden at home by age 38. Still, she didn't let this temper her determination to aid the sick and wounded, and she spent years improving patient care and advocacy from her bed.

She published a book, *Notes on Nursing*, in 1859, which detailed how to successfully run and maintain civilian hospitals in two essays. Due to its success, she was often consulted during America's Civil War on how to effectively manage field hospitals.

Her ideals—compassion, commitment to patient care, and diligent hospital administration—were honored by the Queen of England with an estimated £45,000 prize. Nightingale used the money to build St. Thomas' Hospital in 1860, furthering her cause. Within the hospital, she founded the Nightingale Training School for Nurses, creating the first official training program for the profession. Her mission: to give nurses a streamlined skillset specifically for hospital work.

For her efforts, Nightingale became a figure of public admiration. Thanks to her tireless work, the image of nursing shifted; even women from wealthy backgrounds began to seek admission to the school. At last, nursing was elevated from a role of servitude to a venerable profession, and nurses were granted the recognition they'd long deserved.

. . .

Just as formal training for nurses and doctors was being increasingly institutionalized, the next big shift to hospitals and the medical profession occurred in the 1900s. This eventually permeated all areas of social living. This was a time in history following the Industrial Revolution when the scientific method was being applied to the concept of labor productivity. In *The Principles of Scientific Management*, Frederick Taylor described his scientific assessment of how the management of workers impacted productivity. The goal was to optimize tasks and specializations to create best practices in the workplace.

In *The Principles of Scientific Management*, Taylor observed:

Even in the case of the most elementary form of labor that is known, there is science, and that when the man best suited to this class of work has been carefully selected, when the science of doing the work has been developed, and when the carefully selected man has been trained to work in accordance with this science, the results obtained must of necessity be overwhelmingly greater than those which are otherwise possible.

Taylor conducted studies such as timing a worker's sequence of motions with a stopwatch to scientifically prove the optimal way to complete a task. For example, he determined that to achieve maximal productivity, the ideal weight a worker should lift in a shovel was 21 pounds. This knowledge enabled companies to then provide workers with shovels that were optimized for that 21-pound load. Formal performance measures were implemented. As a result, companies saw a three-fold increase in productivity, and workers were rewarded with pay increases. It was a win-win for all involved, at least from a productivity standpoint.

Taylor's methods changed the outlook of the industrial era, as well as the sentiment of these skilled craftsmen. The method took away much of the autonomy that craftsmen had previously enjoyed in their work. With these newly implemented best practices, importance was given only to efficiency and productivity.

After years of various experiments to determine optimal methods, Taylor proposed four principles of scientific management:

1. Replace rule-of-thumb work practices with a scientific method for every task.

2. Scientifically select, train, and teach each worker rather than passively leaving individuals to train themselves.

3. Ensure that work is being done in accordance with scientifically developed methods.

4. Divide work nearly equally between workers assigned to the same task, and encourage management to establish rules to replace the personal preferences and judgments of the individual worker.

These principles were implemented across many places of employment, and the result was increased productivity in each. Henry Ford, for example, applied Taylor's principles in his automobile factories to much success. Even families began to perform household tasks based on the results of these studies.

The only downside was some initial resistance among workers, who complained that this method increased the monotony of their roles. Ultimately, though, collective productivity took precedence over the subjective preferences of individuals. Scientific management changed the way we worked, and decades later these principles were applied to hospitals and physician practices as well.

Taylor's idea of "a fair day's pay for a fair day's work"—based on his belief that all workers were motivated by monetary reward—took off. If a worker didn't achieve his expected output in a given period, it was decided that he didn't deserve to be paid as much as another worker who was more productive. After the idea was generously implemented in doctors' practices and hospitals, every doctor and hospital service within an individual medical facility is paid the same amount (more or less) when providing the same services and procedures. The fee for an appendectomy, for instance, is the same whether a surgeon is fresh out of training or has 20 years of experience. The more patients a doctor sees in a given day, the more productive he or she is, and thus the more lucrative his or her practice's (or the hospital's) bottom-line will be.

The idea of a price tag for treatment fundamentally changed the culture of medicine. In the past, healers charged patients based on what they thought someone could afford, which allowed appointments to follow a more natural schedule. Transactions were more personal and less rushed, as there was no pre-agreed payment for time spent on the services provided.

. . .

In modern times, everything has a price. Although this idea has allowed commerce to flow with great reliability, one major side effect of such innovation has been the way that price has depersonalized patient-physician interactions. A once-intimate encounter has now become more like a transaction.

Doctors went from owning their own instruments (a guarded privilege that resulted in the tradition of passing down the contents of the iconic "black bag" from father to son or daughter) to using surgical instruments and equipment owned by the hospitals. With Taylor's optimization, the role of the doctor shifted from one of an exclusively skilled artisan to something more systematic, collaborative, and centralized.

As for nursing staff, the once all-encompassing duties of this profession were separated into individual tasks: patient care, housekeeping, and administrative and allied services, such as counseling, social work, and patient advocacy. Standard training programs for each of these distinct roles were established.

While it became a necessity to stratify these tasks into more manageable units, the Industrial Age transformed hospitals into factory-style federations. In present day, the moment a patient is admitted to a hospital, there is a predictable, ritualistic sequence of events that occurs. We use methodical procedures for admittances, ordering tests, obtaining results, following treatment protocols, and processing discharges. With these methods, management teams can measure precisely what the hospital staff is doing and can fine-tune how to complete tasks better, faster, and cheaper. Actions are observed and tracked, outcomes are measured, and procedures and responsibilities are adjusted until productivity increases. Work flow is constantly reorganized—just like factory assembly lines— to achieve maximum efficiency. Workers became compliant cogs in a giant machine, and doctors and nurses were no different.

Despite such corporatization of medical care, nursing training continues to largely emphasize addressing patients' psychosocial issues from a more holistic view. Nursing, which essentially means "to nourish," exemplifies a job that not only involves caring for the sick, aged, and debilitated, but also promotes health and vigor in those who are well. In fact, in order to establish nursing as a distinct profession, much effort has been made to avoid the medical model in nursing training. While still keeping up to date with many of the latest therapies, pharmaceuticals, equipment, and technologies, nursing training tends to avoid pathophysiologic clinical subjects as primary areas of focus. Instead, more attention is given to the psychosocial and social facets of patient care.

Physicians, however, have undergone an ideological makeover, the consequence of a well-orchestrated transformation over the past 300 years that systematically changed the nature of medical training. Their practice has evolved from healing the whole patient and nourishing the individual to healing isolated diseases—salvaging and patching up broken-down parts.

CHAPTER 14

THE UNEXPECTED INTRUDER

The time will come when medicine will
organize itself into an undercover dictatorship.

—BENJAMIN RUSH

In the fall of 2015, my doctor ordered a CT scan of my chest for a chronic, nagging cough I'd been suffering from for close to three months. Although he suspected the cough was the result of an upper respiratory infection, acid reflux, allergies, or a combination of the three, the persistence of my symptoms is what led to the CT recommendation. The scan turned out to be normal, the cough was attributed to seasonal allergies, and in a few days I was back to my usual self. Shortly after my test, I received a letter from my insurance provider. I wasn't surprised to see it, but it piqued my interest all the same. It read:

> This letter is notification regarding the review of clinical information necessary to determine if the tests are medically necessary, as defined in your plan document.
>
> Based on the information submitted, we have determined the recommended test is medically necessary.

What was once left to the sole discretion of a physician is now probed by a third-party agency: the health-insurance provider. In a radical departure from how medicine has been practiced since the beginning of time, neither the dialogue regarding my well-being nor the care path necessary to ensure my health are private matters between my doctor and myself. If my insurance company had rejected the test and refused to pay for the scan, my doctor would have been tasked with appealing the decision. This would involve a lengthy phone call or letter explaining why the tests he ordered were required.

This third-party intervention arose not merely as a payment system but out of social and economic need. It first reared its head when medicine began to take a more scientific approach. The scientific method not only gave the physician tools to understand human physiology, it also did something unexpected: It changed the entire style and substance of how doctors practice medicine.

In general, professions are venerated depending on how uniquely they contribute to the welfare of society. Physicians are cherished not only for their expertise, but also for the admirable ethics to which they adhere. In this case, trust isn't earned, it's assumed. Doctors are reckoned with a level of confidence, perhaps more than any other profession, from the very first encounter they share with their patients. There exists a belief that this individual—by virtue of being a physician—is bound by ethical rules preventing the exploitation of his or her knowledge and skill, a promise rarely unbroken.

Physicians are taught to carry themselves in a particular way. They are expected to be unpretentious toward patients and genuinely devoted to their profession. This expectation is held in close regard, given that their decisions will bear a lasting impact on an irreplaceable entity of nature: the individual's life. Their presence has long assumed a level of superiority—that a patient will accept his or her decision-making without much question.

As late as 1969, the philosopher Hans Jonas asserted that "the physician is obligated to the patient and no one else. . . . We may speak of a sacred trust; strictly by its terms, the doctor is, as it were, alone with his patient and God."

Well into the post-World War II era, bedside decisions were essentially the sole concern of the physician. This was true even when the situation concerned fundamental ethical and social issues. It was exclusively doctors, for instance, who weighed the risks of withholding antibiotics and letting pneumonia bring a fairly swift end to a suffering, declining life. Physicians formed their decisions on a case-by-case basis, responding to a particular circumstance as they saw fit. In turn, the patients and their families almost always heeded the physician's judgment.

Yet by the late 1900s, the untethered authority that an individual physician once exercised was now subject to debate and review by colleagues, law makers, and public opinion. The social and economic transformations that have ensued since are responsible for permanently altering the dynamics of the patient-physician relationship. The primary driver of this change was an age-old nemesis: the cost of medical care.

Throughout the Middle Ages, for example, individuals who fell ill could call a physician. Given the steep fees, however, this service was typically only utilized by the wealthy. Though there were instances of doctors treating the poor for a reduced fee—or even free of charge—these services weren't consistently available.

Dr. John Hall (the son-in-law of William Shakespeare) of Stratford, England (1575–1635), often indicated in his case notes that he tended to the care of all members of a household he visited, servants included. It's assumed that the head of the household covered the cost in those instances, giving rise to the concept of the family physician. Still, this was more of an outlier than the norm.

Less-affluent middle-class families typically relied on an apothecary to provide any medications prescribed by a doctor. The apothecary was also consulted for treatment advice—a role that steadily expanded during this era.

. . .

The relationship between physicians and pharmacists is an interesting alliance that has evolved through centuries. In antiquity, there was no such distinction; priest-physicians also served as pharmacists, dispensing medicines that they prepared themselves. From the earliest times, medicine men of primitive tribes collected herbs and concocted medicinal remedies, the formulas of which were kept secret and passed down within familial circles or to carefully selected apprentices.

For hundreds of years, every aspect of medical care existed entirely within the purview of the physician. Yet as physicians focused more on diagnosis and treatment, one aspect of the medicine man's many skills—preparing and dispensing medications—began to break away from the well-guarded profession.

By the medieval period, it was the monasteries that carried out the dispensing of medicine. In the eighth century, Arabs opened the earliest recorded pharmacy shops. Due to foreign trade routes, dispensaries started to appear in Europe around the eleventh century, with Italy and France leading the trend. The owners of these dispensaries were typically herb and spice traders who later learned to prepare medicinal concoctions as the demand for this skill grew. They came to be called "apothecaries," which literally translates to *shopkeeper*.

Over time, apothecaries strengthened as business entities. They grew to form associations, dispense drugs, and then even to diagnose illnesses and prescribe treatments. Many apothecaries further expanded their roles to include practicing general medicine and sometimes dentistry. As a result, a conflict arose between physicians (who charged more due to their specialized training) and apothecaries (who charged less for medical care while making a profit from the sale and supply of medications, which were prescribed by both parties). Physicians were increasingly disgruntled by the unexpected intrusion of apothecaries into their field, and it became necessary to regulate the profession.

Fredrick II of Hohenstaufen, the emperor of Germany and king of Sicily, was the first to make major strides in this arena. An intelligent ruler with knowledge of philosophy, medicine, and fluency in several languages, he saw the need for clarity between these two competing parties. In 1231, he presented the Edict of Palermo to Sicily and Southern Italy, the primary feature of which separated the two professions as unique fields, each with its own skills, responsibilities, and regulations.

To help prevent the exploitation of those needing medical care, Hohenstaufen ruled that physicians could not own or work in partnership with apothecaries. Further, a list of acceptable drugs for pharmaceutical use was created by the government with some effort to control pricing. Specific drugs were required to be stocked and available and were also given an expiration date of one year, after which they had to be discarded.

It wasn't long before principles of the edict spread across Europe and similar legislation cropped up elsewhere. In addition to the limitations placed on physicians preventing them from dispensing medication in competition with apothecaries, pharmacists were barred from charging for medical consultations. Instead, they had to earn their profits exclusively from the sale of drugs and medications.

Once pharmacists were prohibited from prescribing treatments of their own, those who were too poor for a physician sought medical treatment from members of religious communities if they were available. For centuries, people had been relying on charitable and religious organizations, as well as local associations, which collected or maintained "poor funds" or "sickness funds" for low-income individuals. But there was no guarantee the money from these funds would be available when it was needed most.

By the fourteenth and fifteenth centuries, a few old trade associations developed a system of allocating relief funds through "collecting boxes" for the poor as a way to support members financially if they couldn't pay medical expenses themselves. Travelers, craftsmen, factory workers, and even those who didn't fit into any particular trade were served in this way by guild memberships. These funds became the first type of insurance. They focused mainly on the underprivileged, enabling low-income households to fall back on a more reliable form of relief when illness struck. But these arrangements were poorly enforced and unavailable in many European cities, leaving a majority of the poor with limited access to medical care. Out of desperation, socioeconomically disadvantaged populations became vulnerable to traveling salesmen and con artists advertising cheap cure-alls—a predicament with often dangerous consequences.

By the seventeenth century, governments were in desperate need of an equitable arrangement that would provide medical expenses for those who could not afford care. Little did they know that the implementation of a social-support program would go on to change the entire landscape of the medical profession.

. . .

The Scientific Revolution brought with it experimental medicine and the promise of saving lives using improved medical practice. These experimental methods discredited many healing practices as unscientific or shams, leaving the poor at an even greater disadvantage. Adding to this, the cost of training physicians and running hospitals was a growing burden to the system. The only solution for maintaining these costs was to pass off the rising price tag to the patients in the form of elevated medical expenses. For those who were economically disadvantaged, access to care was becoming increasingly difficult; the poor simply couldn't afford to be ill.

Before we adjusted to these changes, another major transition occurred. The Scientific Revolution, with its newfound knowledge and techniques, spawned the Industrial Revolution, and the West began to transform from an agrarian economy to a mechanized one. From the mid-eighteenth to early-nineteenth century in Europe, hand-production methods were replaced by machines, and employment in factories became the new way of life. Governments needed to incentivize people to take on the resulting high-risk jobs, such as mining and railway construction, while at the same time keeping workers healthy.

This transition didn't come without consequence. Though there was an increase in productivity, there was also a spike in work-related deaths. Accident insurance was the first trialled solution but was far too expensive given the unpredictable nature of such on-the-job accidents. The result was an enormous conflict between insurance providers and beneficiaries.

Governments needed a cost-effective system to provide a livelihood for families who'd lost their sole breadwinner. They were, essentially, searching for a way to determine the monetary value of an individual's life. This concept of estimating someone's projected cost of sickness and death, known today as actuarial science, didn't yet exist.

With the rapidly increasing need to be able to assess personal risk more scientifically, mathematicians came to our rescue again. Eighteenth-century astronomer and mathematician Edmond Halley (a colleague of Newton's and the man of Halley's Comet fame) constructed a mathematical model that could be used to calculate the currency value of future contingent events, such as the mortality rates of a given age. This enabled statisticians to calculate how much money should be set aside to pay for the future death benefits of an insured person. Thus, the idea of a life-insurance policy was born. These mathematical formulas eventually helped develop payment models for the sick and went on to become the healthcare insurance and pension plans we recognize today.

Health insurance was originally restricted to cover only a few major life-changing events, such as pregnancy, loss of limb, or a serious health crisis. Much like the early life-insurance schemes, it was only the governments that provided for health plans. Germany was an early adopter.

Bismarck, the country's "Iron" chancellor, set the tone with his notion that the government must "look after him when he is ill," referring to the factory worker. The concept of the "welfare state" was thus established for the first time in the modern world when Bismarck made it the government's responsibility to provide its citizens with minimal provisions for a good life. While similar ideas had been implemented in the past, they were nothing like Germany's structured system, which was enforced with fierce conviction. By the late nineteenth century, many European governments began to initiate national health insurance programs modeled after Germany's.

These programs grew during the Second World War, when wage and price controls were placed on employers to divert resources to the military and control steep inflation. To compete for workers, companies in North America began to offer health benefits, giving rise to the employer-based insurance system of our current culture. Many private organizations quickly took advantage of this prosperous business model. Private health insurance companies sprouted like mushrooms all over the country. Health insurance systems became widely implemented throughout the rest of the world as well, provided by governments and private organizations in varying combinations.

This shift in who pays for the healthcare expenses of individuals changed not only the dynamics of how healthcare was funded, it also brought about a remarkable change in how services were delivered by the physician. The patient-physician relationship, once a sacred bond, now had an unexpected intruder: the third-party payer.

Once this system was adopted, contractual relationships between the physician and the payer—as well as between the patient and the payer—were established. Physicians were forced to adjust their style of practice. Due to the high stakes—the individual's life—the relationship between the payer and the provider had to be controlled by the government through immense legislation. Working under that contract, the physician was legally and professionally obligated to act in the patient's best interest, while the third-party payer was contractually obligated to pay for services rendered by the physician. These checks and balances have ensured that this arrangement, in theory, continues to benefit and protect all parties involved. Though the overarching goal of insurance remains the same, the intricacies of coverage continue to evolve.

The third-party payers, acting in the interest of the patient (or themselves), have worked to ensure physicians follow established best practices. If a third-party payer determines that a physician strays from professional guidelines and orders tests that are deemed *medically not necessary* through their assessment, for instance, the payer imposes barriers on the physician by way of withholding payment. As a result, physicians are coerced to order services for patients that fall within these third-party-payer guidelines.

The intention behind these ideas was good. Although insurance is still too expensive for many individuals worldwide, a vast majority of people in the modern era have access to medical care they otherwise wouldn't. But the introduction of a regulating element between patient and physician (especially one with its own financial interests) means that both patients and physicians have to adjust to the new ecosystem. The insurance industry has grown to such proportions that it's become a gatekeeper of which tests and services a doctor can order and whom the patient can approach for care. These barriers are an undesirable consequence of a system that's saved more lives than was possible before its inception.

In this triangular relationship, physicians have started to feel like skilled agents of these third-party providers. The paternalistic character once exercised by doctors is now carried out by the insurance providers themselves, detaching physicians emotionally one step further.

CHAPTER 15

MEDICINE'S NEW MYSTICAL FORCE

The physician must be able to tell the antecedents, know the present,
and foretell the future—must mediate these things.

—HIPPOCRATES

Consider a neurologist's thought process when a patient has lost sensation in her feet and is having trouble walking. The doctor is faced with
two challenges: first, identifying the source of the problem; second,
developing a treatment plan.

What caused this? Is the disorder in the feet, in the nerves that carry
sensory impulses, or in the muscles? Is it in the joints of the ankles,
knees, or hips? Or, more alarmingly, might the problem be in the spine
or brain? Is the patient having a stroke that's presenting in an unusual
way? What tests should be ordered? How often should the doctor follow up? The list goes on and on.

How a doctor detects what's wrong with a patient has been the
object of my fascination since I was nine years old. I've always been
curious about the process by which a doctor recognizes what can't be
seen with the naked eye and is then able to prognosticate the outcome

of the disease. This curiosity was the impetus for my interest years later in studying medicine.

Centuries ago, the clinical knowledge and cognitive skills of a medical professional were perceived as a mysterious aptitude, a talent that separated physicians from everyone else. Hacking the human operating system remained exclusively in the hands of doctors. Divination was replaced by observation-based knowledge and reason around 2,000 years ago, yet the ancient impression of a doctor as a sort of prophetic magician who can interpret the mystery of human biology has stuck around ever since.

There's a story from the first century AD when Galen, the most prominent Greek physician of the time, describes meeting a sick person by happenstance and curing him in the street:

> When I encountered one of these [patients suffering from fever] by chance, and he explained that he had recently begun shivering, I stopped the shivering on the spot by giving him bread from diluted wine . . . on the way to my clinic.

Galen was known for showing off his penetrating observational skills and his ability to trace the cause of an illness, like an infallible fortune-teller who could predict the fate of any ill-stricken patient. It's reported that he once walked into a patient's house and, upon seeing the contents of his bedpan—which appeared like "a newly slaughtered meat"—he immediately suspected the disease was of the liver. The patient was being treated for inflammation around the lungs, called pleurisy, with a "concoction of hyssop and honey." Galen, however, attributed the patient's right-sided rib pain to his inflamed liver. Galen was right: The ailment was a foodborne illness from which the patient eventually recovered, and little medical intervention was necessary. This savvy judgment is what ultimately led to the esteem associated with the

art of medicine. For centuries, doctors have enjoyed a special social status due to this particularly unique skillset.

The Arab physician al Razi (AD 841–926) was a doctor and scholar
whose descriptions of diseases rank with those of Hippocrates. Describing a popular perception of physicians, he wrote:

> The physician knows everything and requires to ask no ques-
> tions. If he inspects the urine or feels the pulse, he is supposed
> to know what the patient has and what he has been doing. . . .
> When I began to practice medicine, [I] had resolved to ask no
> questions when the urine had been given to me and had been
> much honored. Later, when it was seen that I made circumstan-
> tial inquiries, my reputation sank.

Even until the 1970s, medical students were told by their instructors
never to open a book in front of a patient. In the event that they didn't
know something, such as the dosage of a drug they were about to prescribe, students were advised to excuse themselves, leave the room, and
look up the information out of sight of the patient. Only then should
they return, continuing on as if they had known the solution all along.

It was thought that in order for physicians to establish credible trust
with patients, this critical component of the therapeutic relationship
was necessary. The patient's expectation was that the physician would
have all of the answers to cure an illness immediately available in memory, and it was the doctor's duty to embody that ideal.

For medical students, the best way to act as if they could truly retain
everything they needed to know was to literally know everything. They
would spend countless hours memorizing the available medical texts,
committing hundreds upon hundreds of pages to memory.

. . .

In ancient healing practices, diagnosis by sensory and extrasensory perception was the medicine man's means to translate the language of biological process. Healers relied on a sort of synesthesia, a muddling of senses, in their attempt to detect maladies because "feeling the spirit" was their primary gateway to diagnosis. The sacred touch of mystics or—as with ancient African traditions—the incantations of indigenous healers were used to form conclusions about illnesses and cures.

By the Middle Ages, identifying an illness became a cognitive process. The practice of relying on sensory knowledge strengthened and proliferated through the Renaissance, a long stretch spanning almost from the sixth to the seventeenth century. The fourteenth-century physician Arnaldus de Villa Nova observed, "All true knowledge arises from the senses." This was in an era when salt was tested by touch and glass was certified by hearing. Physicians felt pulses, smelled plague, and used taste and touch to diagnose diseases.

Complex pattern recognition emerged as the gateway to diagnosis, and doctors relied on their sensory observation of cues from the patient to form an opinion about an illness. In the process, doctors gathered information from several regions of the body. Clinicians' perceptions of what could be felt, what was palpable, and what was visibly noticeable were the only means available to detect an imbalance. Through the evolution of these methods, physicians' perceptive skills became unrivaled as diagnostic tools.

The period of the Scientific Revolution in the seventeenth and eighteenth centuries continued to be typified by physicians' subjective assessments with an even more aggressive pursuit. Physical examination relied on a sequence of highly skilled acts performed by a doctor in an attempt to gain insight into the mechanisms of the biological factory beneath the skin. Their tools were still their senses alone—feeling the pulse or tapping the ribcage. Physicians throughout the Age of Enlightenment were engrossed in mastering subjective skills, which they lovingly called "the bedside diagnosis."

One physician, Josef Leopold Auenbrugger, spent several years at a Spanish hospital perfecting his technique, which allowed him to detect ailments hidden within the thorax.[1] The most illustrious nineteenth-century physician, however, was Pierre Louis, whose writings set the key agenda of new hospital medicine. Graduating in 1813, Louis spent nearly seven years perfecting bedside clinical skills before publishing a number of books and essays on the subject.

Louis's essay "Clinical Instruction" set the standard for French hospital medicine. He regarded a doctor's ability to examine and diagnose patients at the bedside with the highest importance. This skill was considered the best method for identifying diseases. Medical training focused exclusively on instructing students in the techniques of using their senses, whether through touching parts of the body to distinguish subtle changes or training the ears and nose to recognize specific sounds and peculiar smells of disease.

As part of this sensory education, there was an emphasis on developing a strong connection with the patient. Many diagnostic acts involved touching body zones not normally exposed or handled. Touch became a fundamental necessity when examining a patient, and it helped the physician become acquainted with the individual in his or her care. This rapport helped build further trust between patients and physicians.

Around this time, nineteenth-century doctors started to forge bold steps in learning the inside of the human body by augmenting their senses with instruments. Before this, listening to a patient's heart and lungs meant direct application of the doctor's ear to the patient's chest.

---

1   These observations were published in a little book called *Inventum Novum ex Percussione Thoracis Humani Interni Pectoris Morbos Detegendi* (the full English title is *A New Discovery that Enables the Physician from the Percussion of the Human Thorax to Detect the Diseases Hidden Within the Chest*). It is considered a book that marks an epoch in the modern history of medicine.

French physician René Laënnec had particular difficultly with this technique. In 1816, he described this method as "not only ineffective but inconvenient, indelicate and, in hospitals, even disgusting." The practice was especially appalling to Laënnec when he was providing care to female patients. As one writer satirically recounted, "Doctors were known to have laid their heads upon a soft bosom, and in a matrimonial way dropped off to sleep."

Confronted by a young woman who was particularly well endowed, Laënnec tried something new: rolling a piece of paper and listening to her chest from a comfortable distance. Surprisingly, he was able to hear her heartbeat with even greater clarity than the ear-to-chest method. Laënnec spent the next three years testing various tools to improve the ability to listen to the chest of patients with heart and lung diseases, and the stethoscope was born.

With the ability to more clearly distinguish between different breath sounds, Laënnec was able to diagnose many lung ailments, including bronchitis, pneumonia, and pulmonary tuberculosis. Yet despite growing assistance from tools and instruments, physicians during this era continued to rely on direct sense perception, and their training was geared toward honing these abilities. So much emphasis was placed on perfecting bedside clinical techniques that therapeutics remained subordinate to diagnostic skills.

One consequence of this was that physicians were adept at identifying many diseases they had no idea how to cure. Many doctors still relied on the concept of the healing power of nature—the ability of the body to restore itself to health. For instance, by the end of the nineteenth century, physicians knew for sure that diabetes was the result of a higher -than-normal amount of sugar in the body, but they were stumped as far as treatment was concerned. At the time, the average life expectancy of a 10-year-old child with diabetes was only about a year. A diagnosis at age 30 carried only a slightly higher life expectancy of about four years.

By the mid-twentieth century, physicians had rapidly upgraded their clinical expertise by inventing instruments to help detect illnesses. With the use of scopes and scans, reliance on subjective assessment began to take a backseat to measurement and quantification. Still, for centuries this practice remained the primary means of identifying abnormalities.

The young physicians-in-training were taught vigorously to perfect the skills of bedside diagnosis, while reliance on technology was frowned upon in academic circles. Master clinician Joseph D. Sapira elaborately described these skills in *The Art and Science of Bedside Diagnosis*, published in 1989. In determining heart diseases, for instance, Sapira directs physicians to perfect the art of listening to the heart and evaluating each organ system through careful observation. Most importantly, doctors were tasked with learning how to listen for an extended period of time without making the patient quiver, thinking that something must be terribly wrong.

To teach these skills, Sapira would tape-record clinical interviews between patients and medical students. Then, together with each student, he would listen to the tapes. Using a stopwatch, he would time the period between the end of a patient's answer and the beginning of the student's next question. His goal was to teach future physicians how to create longer pauses to ensure they'd get the best information from the patient and thus be able to accurately classify the problem.

Sapira instructed his students to tell patients at the beginning of an auscultation of the heart: "I may listen to your heart for a long time. This doesn't mean I am hearing anything bad." He advised budding doctors to "remember that the patient will be observing your facial expressions but that you will not be attending to his responses as you concentrate on what you are auscultating." Sapira's first rule was that doctors must listen in a completely quiet room.

Being painstakingly taught by physicians who were trained in medical schools during the 1960–70s, I imbibed certain professional routines myself, one of which was bedside diagnosis—now a dwindling skill. My professors believed in the dictum that what makes a doctor exceptional is how he or she uses physical examination practices to arrive at a diagnosis, and they instilled this notion in us.

. . .

Early in my training, I had a 61-year-old male patient who was being evaluated for a stroke that left him weak on his left side. A nursing student noticed an irregular pulse and called me to take a look. The patient described feeling a sensation as if his heart was skipping a beat, something he'd never experienced before. Resting comfortably, the patient reached out his right hand for me. His pulse was indeed irregular. This was only the second day of my rotations during my intern year, so experience was not on my side. A sincere student, I quickly began applying my training to diagnose the abnormal pulse.

The exact character of the pulse was vital to determine whether or not the patient needed to be on blood-thinning medication for the rest of his life. This could not be a snap decision. I spent about a few minutes meticulously trying to feel the pulse as it erratically hit my fingers. Then I listened to the heartbeat with utmost attention, after which I reported my findings to my senior resident who was swamped with a heavy patient load. I spurted out what I thought to be all of the necessary information I'd observed. As politely as he could, the resident fired back: "Why don't you get an EKG? We have so many patients we still need to check before the morning rounds in 10 minutes." *Of course*, I realized. An EKG, which is a tracing of electrical activity of the heart, is the easiest way to diagnose an irregular heart rhythm. Why hadn't I thought to do this? Such a major decision couldn't be left to my guesswork.

In my medical school days, there was a sense of pride in being able to make a correct diagnosis using only our clinical skills while with a patient.

How Doctors Diagnosed Ilnesses Across Time

ANTIQUITY
1300 BC–AD 500

Medicine men use occult powers to diagnose illnesses. They touch patients to connect to the soul. The village healer is a mystic with no objective proof of his conclusions.

MEDIEVAL AGE
AD 500–AD 1450

Clues from a person's history are the primary gateway to diagnosis. Physicians rely on observation, such as the visual examination of bodily fluids and feeling the patient's pulse.

RENAISSANCE
AD 1450–AD 1650

Diagnosis at bedside gains importance. Touching patients instills trust in doctors. The art of medicine dominates the profession.

AGE OF ENLIGHTENMENT
AD 1650–AD 1800

Scientific methods help physicians test the validity of their bedside assessments. More illnesses are diagnosed at bedside, but treatments lag behind.

AGE OF INNOVATION
AD 1800–AD 1920

Instruments are invented to aid in bedside diagnosis, such as the stethoscope and thermoscope. Bedside diagnosis matures, and physicians value it as the most important skill of their profession.

AGE OF INSTRUMENTS
AD 1920–AD 2000

Utilizing technology like scans, EKG, and X-rays becomes the norm. Doctors increasingly use instruments to test and diagnose, relying less on bedside diagnosis.

AGE OF INFORMATION
1980–21st CEN.

Doctors' knowledge about the human body grows exponentially using scientific methods. Bedside conclusions become even less reliable as disease-centered diagnosis moves from physicians to machines.

AGE OF AUTOMATION
21st CEN.–FUTURE

Dominance of technology aides diagnosis and treatment to push doctors into a symbiotic role with machines. Physicians also assume more supportive roles, such as patient counselor.

To identify a murmur required several hours of intense training through observation, not to mention years of trial and error to master this art. As students, we were tasked with identifying the location, intensity, pitch, and radiation of a murmur—listening to the chest during inspiration, expiration, squatting, sitting, standing, lying, bending forward, leaning forward, and during breath-holding. By the time I was in practice, these and most other bedside skills were far less relevant.

As the twenty-first century marches on, many of these abilities are on the decline. Our idea of bedside diagnosis is like attempting to measure a patient's temperature using a palm to the forehead. With technology at our fingertips, there's no reason to speculate. The assurance and accuracy of technology is clearly better.

With so many treatment options, doctors were no longer able to rely on memorization. The seemingly infinite realms of options made it impossible to keep track of all of the potential interactions and side effects of these drugs.

Not all physicians were pleased with this shift in their routine; reliance on algorithms and protocols is less satisfying to those physicians who pride themselves on bedside diagnostic skills and rely on expert opinions as preferred methods of medical practice.

The argument against these algorithms is that they encourage doctors to focus on numbers. Herbert L. Fred of the University of Texas Health Science Center, a professor of internal medicine, believes that algorithms lead physicians to interact with numbers, not patients, and has urged medicine to "give algorithms back to the mathematicians." Just like the eighteenth-century physicians who resisted the application of statistics to medicine, there are physicians who continue to resist the introduction of technology and a protocol-based approach to medicine.

Here's an example of the good work formalized protocols can do: Chemotherapy drugs, first introduced in the 1940s, are selected based on a variety of information and factors. The treatment has undergone decades of investigations; clinical trial after clinical trial has been conducted to standardize the treatment and compile best practices. Through relentless study, specific protocols involving the medications, doses, and schedule based on the type and stage of the cancer have been determined.

The most important metric used to measure the success of different chemotherapy treatments is what's known as the response rate. This is the number of people whose tumors have shrunk or disappeared as a result of taking these drugs. If certain types and stages of cancer have a 65 percent response rate to a certain combination of drugs, for instance, this means that 65 percent of people suffering from that type and stage of cancer would respond to treatment, whereas 35 percent wouldn't have a noticeable response.

Along with these rates, response durations are analyzed by other metrics, such as how long the responses will last. Based on these protocols, oncologists choose treatments with the highest response rates and longest known durations.

A chemotherapeutic drug isn't to be taken lightly; it's loaded with risks due to its toxic nature. The health of an individual is yet another factor a doctor must take into consideration for chemo cocktails. For those who are frail, elderly, or suffering multiple ailments, the benefit may not be worth the risk, leaving oncologists to focus instead on simply ensuring quality of life.

There isn't one correct choice for chemotherapy. Each protocol bears its own unique blend of advantages and disadvantages, and protocols are always evolving as more data proves value or ineffectiveness. Even with all factors considered, the treatment that should theoretically achieve maximum response rates sometimes fails, and no matter how hard we try, there's no way to predict the outcome of therapy for any individual. The point is that these algorithms lead oncologists through the complicated maze of complex treatment options for life-threatening illnesses.

This is true for a range of other drugs and treatments as well. Ultimately, the only thing that matters is how precisely a doctor can diagnose an illness and develop an appropriate treatment plan, by whatever means necessary. Subjective assessment in the form of bedside clinical skills is still indispensable and in certain situations can be useful. Professionals who can benefit from them include field medics in the armed services, doctors practicing medicine in developing countries where technology is less available or where necessities like electricity aren't guaranteed, and EMTs and first responders in developed nations who need to make assessments and medical decisions without the convenience of hospital equipment.

The subjective judgment of a physician, once an exalted aptitude, is now seen as inadequate and liable to error. Objective proof has become imperative for accurate diagnosis and in order to standardize care. Simply feeling that my patient had an irregular pulse was not enough to plan treatment. Instead, I had to order an objectively verifiable test. If I suspect stroke, there's MRI; for appendicitis, there's CT scan; for heart attack, we have angiogram. Through the application of scans, ultrasounds, and endoscopes, technology has allowed doctors to "see" inside of our patients' bodies, thereby improving the accuracy of our diagnoses.

. . .

As physicians acquire relevant information from patients through interviews, physical exams, lab tests, and other investigations, they routinely use shortcuts to quickly assess and arrive at a diagnosis, weeding through copious possible options. Each piece of information becomes part of a probability analysis to help determine the odds that a fever is due to sinusitis and not meningitis, for instance. If one piece does not fit the clinical conundrum, the doctor restructures the problem and switches from shortcuts to elaborate mental maps, developing detailed outlines of relevant tests and treatments to unlock the mystery.

As doctors gain more and more experience, they can—in some ways—get slower over the years in certain areas and faster in others. They know more about the mistakes they make and thus try to do things carefully enough to avoid them, which can slow them down. They now also know more and can shortcut many more tasks that were formerly time consuming, which can speed them up. The cerebral process that takes place inside a well-trained doctor's head is astonishing.

This is not to say that no personal bias enters into decision-making. To the contrary, plenty of research proves that doctors looking at the same issue will disagree with each other 10 to 50 percent of the time in many areas of care, from performing a physical examination to interpreting a laboratory test to recommending a treatment. This variable nature of physician judgment is highly endemic. In his acclaimed book *How Doctors Think*, Jerome Groopman enumerates numerous studies on this inconsistency within various medical specialties. Even the most competent doctor is liable to error because of the nature of the field. Sometimes clinical conditions prove to be a hard nut to crack. Human biology, being inherently variable, sets limits on our reasoning and unveils our vulnerability.

As we dig deeper into the mysteries of our own biology, we're faced with a counterintuitive phenomenon that our ancient and medieval healers could never have conceptualized: The more experience a physician accumulates, the more out-of-date some aspects of his or her practice are likely to become. Research shows that the quality of clinical performance decreases as years in practice increase. Contrary to the general assumption that the more knowledge and skills physicians accumulate, the better patient outcomes will be, those physicians may paradoxically be *less* likely to provide the most effective treatments.

David Sackett, widely regarded as "the Father of evidence-based medicine," gained notoriety in the medical community for repeating his residency in medicine some 20 years after first training. Though he was already a professor in the medical school, he felt he "wasn't a good enough doctor." The reason for this is that doctors tend to become married to more antiquated methods over time, including many that were handed down by their mentors.

Modern doctors—who once were able to pick treatment options based solely on what they were taught during their training—are now faced with information overload. Innovation has begun to outpace students' abilities to learn and memorize. The rate of advancement, coupled with growing efficiencies of mass production, means that more choices are now at a physician's disposal. Consider diabetes, for which insulin was the only medication used in the 1920s, but today has eight different classes of medications available for treatment. Over the next decade, it's anticipated that we'll develop more than 180 new drugs to treat diabetes and its related conditions.

To avoid inconsistencies and aid physicians as they dig through mountains of information, the medical community came up with a solution in the last decade of the twentieth century. It would employ standardized algorithms to ensure that every doctor uses similar thought processes, thus providing a way for treatments to be systematized and standardized. These algorithms—cognitive maps between symptoms and diagnoses—are based on research and are agreed upon by experts in each field.

Protocols surrounding these algorithms serve as mental guideposts for physicians, aiding in both how to arrive at a diagnosis and how to treat an ailment. Protocols these days run the routines of medical practices, from proper hand-scrubbing techniques to hospital waste disposal to managing trauma patients. A surgeon's routine in the operating room is strictly protocol-based as well. So are all of the important activities that take place in intensive care units. A patient rushed into the emergency department with a gunshot injury to the neck that's sliced major blood vessels, for example, can trigger a frenzy if not handled systematically.

Healthcare teams are prone to omissions in ordering the right tests, missteps in administering the correct medications, and potential judgment errors due to the stresses of dealing with life-threatening situations. Computerized protocols systematize these processes and make for objective assessment and fool-proof mechanisms, with tight checks and balances along the way. There's no room left for guesswork.

Medical knowledge and cognitive decision-making, once the sole proprietorship of physicians and the mystical force that separates physicians from the rest of us, have been exposed through only a few clicks on a screen.

PART SIX

THE FUTURE DOCTOR

"In the future, a further separation of medicine into two fields—
art and science—is going to become more visible."

CHAPTER 16

TRANSCENDING LIMITATIONS

> The philosophies of one age have become the absurdities of the next, and
> the foolishness of yesterday has become the wisdom of tomorrow.
>
> —SIR WILLIAM OSLER

Our ancient physicians hypothesized many theories based on their observation of human interaction with nature. Most of their theories were rightfully based on seeing an organism as inseparable from its environment. This led to the holistic and personalized approach to an individual's care. These observations eventually became the principles that medical knowledge was built upon.

What they didn't have was a method to test their theories. Even if they had, they would have needed a testable hypothesis. But the concept of humoral balances or energy equilibrium within the human body was not a readily testable hypothesis.

For a modern medical practitioner, there is no room for philosophy or speculation in routine practice. Any medical treatment, drug, or procedure is the outcome of an approach that rests on these four pillars:

1. Experimentation of a proposed idea (hypothesis) in controlled conditions.

2. Population statistics—extracting insights from a few and asserting its truth across a wider population.

3. Intelligent application of the results of the analysis into clinical practice.

4. Constantly testing and re-testing to validate our current practices.

This is the act of science—following these four steps in order to test a hypothesis. Any inquiry that doesn't pass through this grind is simply not grounded in science—it is, at best, a brilliant observation and at worst, a superstition.

Compare this to the fifteenth-century version. Swiss philosopher and physician Paracelsus, who is credited with founding the discipline of Toxicology, defined four pillars of medicine as philosophy, astrology, alchemy, and virtue. Faith and medicine went hand in hand. This shows the drastic shift of how we've approached medicine over time.

Today, all guidelines and policies concerning an individual or community's health should be based on evidence from well-designed and conducted research, not just the observations of practitioners or experts.

The entire body of knowledge in medicine is the product of a specific methodology. In this approach, the subject matter is studied under limited and restricted conditions. In order for us to measure, for instance, a chemical in a test tube with accuracy, we must isolate it from the external environment. Otherwise, even a passing breeze might disturb the results of the analysis. A subtle alteration of temperature might affect the outcome. More and more, we have to isolate the specimen in an influence-proof room. And only then can we have some approximation of the reality. To pretend to be able to do this in human biology seems absurd.

We know that each individual is the interplay of so many known and unknown variables—our eating habits, temperaments, sleep patterns, age, muscle and bone composition, weight, how we metabolize the food we eat, the drugs we take, and so on. Now multiply just this short list of variables alone by even 10,000 individuals in a given population. With a seemingly infinite-sized data set and so many variables to factor in, it's impossible to determine how a drug will affect a particular individual. Even in using the most advanced mathematical and statistical models, no researcher can study the effect of a particular drug over the lifetime of an individual. This is the most difficult problem of life sciences, and measuring changes at this level of complexity creates inherent limitations of our experimental studies.

Yet advancements in human biology will never take place if researchers wait for the perfect conditions to study a new drug or test a cure for a deadly disease. At the same time, it's also impossible to effectively study a biological function that's constantly influenced by so many external factors. To decode the human operating system, we needed to make some concessions.

The entire body of knowledge of a doctor rests on two such fundamental compromises. The first of those is that the laws of chemistry and physics are identical in the world of living things and in that of inanimate matter, as asserted by nineteenth-century physiologist Claude Bernard.

Although it's obvious that the blood in our body and blood in a test tube will not exhibit identical properties, the physiochemical activities in the human body were treated no differently than a set of chemical reactions studied in laboratories under controlled conditions. This crude approximation was a necessity to explore the mechanisms of bodily functions without relying on myth and speculation.

The natural extension of this thought process is to tightly control the variables under study, just like physicists and chemists, which brings us to the second compromise that the scientific medical community collectively agreed to accept.

Because a researcher cannot study all variables at once, they will select only the variable of interest (for instance, the effect of a new drug on blood sugar). All other variables (like the effect of diet, cultural influences, sleep habits, body weight, age, ethnicity, mood changes, etc.) are often assumed constant. This then allows the researcher to focus solely on one factor, such as how a drug affects blood sugar. If these variables aren't assumed constant, then an effort is made to keep the conditions as constant as possible, such as limiting subject participation by age, gender, health, geographic location, or medical history. The time span of studies is also strictly limited to a few months or, at most, a few years.

Every aspect of a disease process is therefore studied in isolation and in controlled lab experiments, then linked to related processes to explain a much bigger functioning.

What this means is that the experimenter is not merely observing, but is actively intervening and altering the natural disease process to understand it through a piecemeal approach. In the words of Claude Bernard, "An experiment is an investigation of natural phenomenon altered by the investigator."

In addition to controlling variables, the experimenter might also utilize a method called randomization. Introduced by the eminent statistician R.A. Fisher in 1935, this method became a historical success in the field of experimental biology. Randomized controlled trials were the new gold standard in large experimental designs, downgrading all other methods to quasi-experiments.

As Fisher noted, the randomization "relieves the experimenter from the anxiety of considering innumerable causes by which the data may be disturbed." The popularity of this approach has been driven largely by its ability to control for known and unknown factors while shielding from external influences that may considerably limit the study process.

. . .

In our experimental approach to studying human biology, the intricate tapestry is being taken apart strand by strand. Each piece is separated and analyzed. But when scientists try to put the pieces back together, they recognize that the whole seems much more elusive than the sum of its parts. Human biology is not simply an aggregate of different mechanisms that can be comprehended using chemical equations and physical laws.

As Erwin Schrodinger, a Nobel-Prize-winning Austrian physicist and pioneer of Quantum physics, observed in *What Is Life*:

> The arrangements of the atoms in the most vital parts of an organism and the interplay of these arrangements differ in a fundamental way from all those arrangements of atoms which physicists and chemists have hitherto made the object of their experimental and theoretical research. . . . The structure of the vital parts of living organisms differs so entirely from that of any piece of matter that we physicists and chemists have ever handled physically in our laboratories or mentally at our writing desks.

Seventeenth-century Western medical practitioners recognized that the key to advancing medical science was to acknowledge the inherent limitation. Personalized medicine simply wasn't a scalable option. This is how the experimental method was born in the West and spread to the rest of the world. It was this particular approach that led your doctor into the current paradigm of treating illnesses rather than treating the complete human being—the disease-centered approach as opposed to a more personalized approach that our ancients tightly held to their hearts but failed to execute. If you ever wondered why your physician treats your illness and not *you*, this is the reason.

The controlled experimental method has proven itself to be of immense value, both in how we treat and prevent many illnesses. But in conceiving this method and then declaring that from henceforth it's the only way to ascertain the truth, we fail to remind ourselves of the limitations inherent to the experimental approach. In fact, we became so fascinated by this approach we forgot to acknowledge that it's designed only to test hypotheses that can be tested in controlled conditions.

This problem is resolved only if we can conceive a method to study our biological processes, not outside the human body, but within, in real time. And not based on population statistics, but individualized data analysis taking into consideration the innumerable variables, including environmental influences that the individual is subjected to.

In other words, our studies should shift from lab to body, from population statistics to individual-specific studies. This is the only way we can transform our current disease-centered approach to a more personalized approach. But we need a system that is so advanced, so powerful that it has to catch the changes happening in our innards and broadcast them live without disturbing the intricate biological architecture. We need a paradigm shift in how we study ourselves.

Medicine's Big Shift
—Technology brings us full circle, restoring personalized care

While the scientific revolution of the seventeenth century introduced a radical change in our thinking, the twenty-first century's digital revolution can be seen as a change in gears of how effectively and efficiently we solve problems.

Holistic Healing

- Religion and medicine go hand-in-hand.
- Theories based largely on observation, opinion, philosophy, and myth.
- Therapeutics involved humoral balances and energy equilibrium.
- Individual-centered approach.

17TH CENTURY SCIENTIFIC REVOLUTION

Disease-Centered Medicine

- Medicine separates from religion and dogma.
- Treatment guidelines based on evidence from controlled experiments and population stats.
- Focus shifts from the individual to diseases.

Personalized Medicine

- Technology broadcasts internal data in real time.
- Shift of population statistics to personalized data.
- Doctors focus on emotional needs and assist in decision-making while treatments are driven by technology.

21ST CENTURY DIGITAL REVOLUTION

MAN-MACHINE SYMBIOSIS

> I keep dreaming of a future, a future with a long and healthy
> life, not lived in the shadow of cancer but in the light.
>
> —PATRICK SWAYZE

I was flying to Boston to attend a medical conference in the spring of
2015 when we were delayed after boarding. The captain announced
that he needed clearance from the ground engineers for a minor problem that had been detected during the standard diagnostics performed
before takeoff. As I sat in my seat watching the bustling airport through
my window, the announcement smacked me with the undeniable recognition that my job as a doctor wasn't much different from how the
ground engineers and pilots ran the plane.

Years ago, when jet engines were adopted by commercial airline companies, they were incredibly complex systems; they were grounded for
preventative maintenance every 125 flight hours, or approximately once
every six months. Monitoring systems relied on hundreds of sensors
placed in various locations within an aircraft engine to gather information about its performance—its "vital signs"—which provided real-time

information to pilots and ground engineers. The moment something varied from the norm, the plane was taken down to pre-empt possible catastrophe.

For airplanes, it was the coming together of sensors and real-time monitoring that made flying more efficient, less expensive, and increasingly accessible. And this approach was also a perfect model for tracking biological changes in the human body. Once unimaginable—just like flight monitoring systems—technological developments like these will continue to empower doctors with an unprecedented assessment of biological processes in real time.

Currently, a majority of our vital measurements are taken in a doctor's office or in hospital labs and radiology departments. Very soon, technology and market forces will converge at the point where sensors have become more accurate and algorithms have grown sophisticated enough to record ongoing, real-time measurements of our vital parameters outside of a hospital or clinic. Wearable and implantable devices are poised to accurately and continuously measure heart rate, blood sugar, oxygen saturation, respiratory rate, blood pressure, and sleep patterns.

Wearable biosensors or peripheral devices (like a blood pressure cuff or pulse oximeter) gather key vitals from a patient and then wirelessly communicate that information to the patient, a third-party monitor, or a team of medical professionals. This information enables more successful daily care and improves preventative measures.

When patients are empowered through these devices to manage their own health, outcomes improve dramatically. Remote communication through telehealth tools aids physicians in staying informed regarding patient health issues, reaching diagnoses, and providing certain types of follow-up care.

Chronic diseases would be more easily supervised and managed, and patients who are too ill or too far away to easily travel could have greater access to care. When the Centers for Disease Control and Prevention took a look at noncritical emergency room visits in a 2011 study, they found that 80 percent of adult patients sought noncritical care at the ER because they lacked access to a primary care physician. In the United States, 60 million people (nearly one in five) don't have regular access to a primary care physician. Remote patient monitoring (RPM) and tele-health technology helps change that.

As this technology grows more ubiquitous, we'll begin to see that doctors aren't the only ones using it to make treatment decisions. Patients will continue to become more involved as they're granted greater access to the data and analytics provided by RPM devices. This will enable them to arrive at appointments with their own body's performance statistics handy. The ability to wirelessly transmit critical patient information will continue to lead to integration with our smartphones through health apps, meaning that we'll essentially be able to carry around a miniature server equipped with our vitals, perhaps even including information as in-depth as the sequence of our entire genomes.

We're working to detect our own bodies' internal sophistication and enhance our abilities to preempt potential misfires—no differently than how we monitor airplanes. And this is just the beginning. In the future, technology is going to assume more of the tasks currently performed by physicians and surgeons, continually changing the style and substance of medicine as we know it today.

Surgeons are already starting to rely on 3D mapping of our internal anatomy well before they ever make the first incision, a capability that helps them anticipate potential mishaps and minimize complications. Surgeons can now perform operations while seated in consoles as they control robots that convert their hands into precision instruments, guided by multiple cameras that provide an unprecedented view inside the body.

Even more impressively, researchers from Washington DC's Children's National Health System started testing their Smart Tissue Autonomous

Robot (STAR) surgical technology, which doesn't depend on a doctor's manual capability. STAR was developed to apply stitches with the same level of skill as top surgeons, all through the use of a 3D imaging system and precise touch sensors—all on its own. In trials on living pigs, the robot stitched with such submillimeter precision that it outperformed its human teachers.

For now, robotic surgery in hospitals is still controlled remotely by a human surgeon and is available for only a select cohort of operations. But with more than 45 million soft-tissue surgeries performed each year in the US, it won't be long before this method becomes the norm, thus eradicating the previous leverage of dexterity that separated a good surgeon from a great one. Surgery is—and increasingly will be—no longer limited by human cognition, coordination, or sight.

Yet robots, much like their human creators, aren't exempt from the possibility of error. There have been reports filed in the last few years documenting surgeries in which the operating robot, controlled by a surgeon at the other end of a console, has nicked blood vessels or clamped down on internal tissue and refused to let go until an entire system reboot has taken place. Still, the benefits appear to outweigh the risks. In a recent study examining a group of patients with prostate cancer, one group received gland-removal surgery by a human surgeon, while another group received the same surgery by a human-controlled robotic surgeon. After three months of recovery, both groups were doing equally well. Patients who had their surgery performed by a robot, however, experienced less blood loss during the procedure, were discharged earlier from the hospital, felt less pain a week after the surgery, and—at six weeks post-op—reported a better physical quality of life.

For Denise Parker, a 54-year-old mother and grandmother, it was a robot that ultimately saved her life. While on a vacation, Parker sought emergency care for what she thought was a bad case of food poisoning. In reality, doctors discovered a cancerous tumor growing in one of her kidneys. She was booked for immediate surgery at London's Guy's and St. Thomas' Hospital. The da Vinci Xi robot, controlled by urological surgeon Ben Challacombe, excised Parker's cancerous right kidney and carefully removed it from Parker's body via a small keyhole incision. Though by this time Dr. Challacombe had performed over 400 partial or complete kidney extractions using the da Vinci, this particular procedure made waves because it was live-streamed for the world to see. Parker's family watched the surgery in real time through the hospital's Twitter feed.

Dr. Challacombe credits the robot with allowing him to work faster, more precisely, and less invasively. And it's true: Denise Parker walked out of the hospital, tumor-free.

Physicians aren't defined any more by the stethoscope, and for a sound reason. The stethoscope, like the knee hammer, is losing its relevance as a critical diagnostic instrument. Physicians are becoming less and less dependent on manual tools. In fact, continual breakthroughs in medicine are allowing us to reach previously concealed recesses of our mortal parts.

Researchers from McGill University, Université de Montréal, and Polytechnique Montréal have been hard at work on a new breakthrough in cancer research: nanorobots that invade the cells of cancerous tumors via the bloodstream, delivering medication directly to target sites. The nanorobots travel from the injection site of a patient through flagellated, self-propelling bacteria, which contain cancer-fighting drugs. The nanorobots detect hypoxic areas—spots in the tumors that lack oxygen—and deliver powerful medication in precise locations to keep the surrounding healthy tissues and organs intact.

And as nanorobot technology improves, our treatment options could expand. Imagine if we could completely eradicate breast cancer, the second-leading cause of cancer deaths in women worldwide. Rather than using today's standard treatments of chemotherapy, radiation, and surgical removal of breast tissue, or even shrinking tumors through targeted nanorobotic delivery, what if the cure was achieved by sending in miniature robots to repair the exact diseased gene responsible for illness? One day, we're going to tackle diseases by the very genes known to cause them. Eventually, this and other technological advancements will be available on a massive scale, elongating our lifespans. By the next century, centenarians will become the norm.

Our ultimate aim is to do the unthinkable—to prolong our youth, the best part of our lives. The philosopher's stone, which our ancient and medieval alchemists labored to discover, will see its fruition by way of technology.

One such cutting-edge development is occurring in transplant technology and regards the ability to transport living organs from donor to recipient. Rather than freezing organs and racing against the clock to deliver them to a waiting patient, strides have been made using a device called Organ Care System (OCS). This system utilizes oxygen and the donor's blood to create a portable environment where the organ continues to function throughout the entire transport process. Though OCS is still in the investigative stage of development, transplant teams at Ronald Reagan UCLA Medical Center used it to transport a beating heart to a donor in 2011. The following year, they successfully delivered a pair of "breathing" lungs to a 57-year-old patient suffering from pulmonary fibrosis.

Capabilities continue to improve, not only in how we transport organs for transplant, but in *what* we transplant. In 2005, a team in France performed the first successful partial-face transplant on Isabelle Dinoire, replacing lower portions of her face after she was mauled by her dog. Five years later, a team of 30 doctors at the Henri-Mondor Hospital in France completed the first successful full face transplant to an anonymous recipient who was disfigured after a shooting accident. In 2012, a transplant team lead by Dr. Eduardo D. Rodriguez at the

University of Maryland Medical Center in the United States pulled off the most extensive full facial transplant to date, giving Richard Norris, also the victim of a firearm accident, an entirely new face after a grueling 36-hour surgery.

As technology continues to improve, more groundbreaking surgical possibilities remain on the horizon. For instance, if an organ or tissue becomes damaged, it's possible that we'll begin to see these parts genetically engineered or grown from healthy cells in labs and replaced surgically. The race is already underway—early in 2016 it was reported that researchers at Wake Forest Baptist Medical in North Carolina used a 3D printer to create bone fragments and successfully implanted them into the bodies of rats. Five months later, the fragments were still thriving and had matured into working tissue with a system of nerves and blood vessels.

In the future, our own skin could be grown or 3D printed if a graft for a third-degree burn is needed. Kidney dialysis machines will one day become the size of current-day insulin pumps. Eventually, biosynthetically grown organ replacement will render even those completely obsolete. The national registry for organ donation may soon become a thing of the past.

Many of these advancements are already happening at the research level, and some of them are being used in clinics and hospitals throughout the world. We'll see their full potential when economies of scale allow such technologies to spread to every part of the globe and become the new standard of care.

. . .

In the current state of technology in medicine, there's an endemic uneasiness among many twenty-first-century medical practitioners. Doctors want the precision that technology affords alongside the ability to use their honed bedside clinical skills. We want to see ourselves as indispensable as we were 100 years ago.

Physicians with this view tend to think the same way our predecessors did when the automation of factories took place in the beginning of the twentieth century. Computerization, though, is not like automation; it is a much more intelligent process. While automation largely replaced blue-collar workers, computerization replaces white-collar workers, too. Automation simply replaced physical labor, but computerization will augment and supplant human intellect.

Because of this, in many ways, technology is seen by some practitioners as a threat to the humanistic side of medicine. Computerization is viewed as something that will potentially erode the sacred doctor-patient relationship.

Consider one increasingly popular use of technology that is the new norm in hospitals: electronic medical records (EMR). Digital health records often contain a person's entire medical history, including their medications and immunization dates, known allergies, lab results, images and scans, and other important information in a single, accessible place. For patients who don't have consistent access to care, or for those who have a long or complex medical history that requires coordination of care from multiple specialists, digital record-keeping can become lifesaving.

Electronic records enable access during times of chaos and disaster. In 2005, when Hurricane Katrina ravaged parts of Louisiana, electronic records were being used for only around 38 percent of patients. Paper records, commonly stored in basements and ground floors of buildings, sat in dirty water or mud for weeks following the storm's devastation.

At the Medical Center of Louisiana in New Orleans, Health Information Supervisor Dorothy Jones prepared for the storm by moving the bottom rows of medical records to a higher shelf in the facility's basement-level storage. When the levee broke, flood water filled the building to the ceiling of the first floor, stranding Jones and many of her colleagues. They were evacuated by boat two weeks later, but the hospital never recovered. Every record was lost. In all, it's estimated that more than 400,000 records from New Orleans-area medical facilities were destroyed in the aftermath of the hurricane.

The impact of this loss was far-reaching. In an interview with ABC News, Dr. Jay Brooks, chief of hematology/oncology at Ochsner Health System in Baton Rouge, Louisiana, recalled seeing New Orleans refugees who didn't know what kinds of medication they were prescribed, what type of cancer they had, or which treatments they'd received.

Digital records are a positive development, but there's a flip side to this technology. In my years working as a medical professional, I've watched a growing number of doctors stay for one to two hours after the work day is finished, come in on days off, or work late at night from home in order to complete the ever-increasing documentation required of the EMR system.

Weary after a long day or night on the job, nurses sift through notes, charts, orders, and Code Blue records. They wade through page-long lists of checkboxes and entry fields asking for descriptive details of what happened in the chaos of an 8-or-12-hour shift, during which they were expected to function simultaneously as caregivers and data-entry clerks.

If the charting system is so labor-intensive, so counterintuitive to the work we do that it can't be successfully used in real time, then shouldn't it be replaced with something better?

I'm not talking about the reality that, of course, some clinicians will chart more slowly or thoroughly than others. This issue goes far beyond that. When a system consistently causes good and efficient medical professionals to stay long past their shifts, or come in on days off, or chart from their homes (which should be places of recuperation and rest), then we need to acknowledge that perhaps there are flaws in the process.

Doctors and nurses rightfully feel that their jobs are to care for people, not to spend hours documenting and charting. As the popularity of EMR systems has increased, this extra workload has seen rampant growth across the profession.

Craig Lambert, a former editor at *Harvard Magazine*, has a name for these added-on responsibilities: shadow work. Any task that isn't done for its own pleasure and that is in some way completed "in the service of an institutional master," falls into this category. For Lambert, shadow work isn't just "a marginal nuisance snipping spare moments away from the edges of life," but rather "a fire-breathing dragon, operating 24/7 throughout." Medical staff, like professionals in many industries, feel that they're tasked with this kind of work—tasks that are necessary, even critical, to their jobs but that don't count directly toward their remuneration.

In 1930, English economist John Maynard Keynes predicted that by 2028 our technology would permit us to work 15-hour weeks and dedicate our lives to leisure. Not even remote signs of such emancipation from toil have happened yet. In fact, it seems to be worsening.

The amount of time spent on clinical documentation has been on the rise since the late 1980s. While electronic records are easier to read, significantly more time is spent on them than on paper charts. And in truth, patients don't like them much, either. A study in *JAMA* found that patients rated the care they received lower when doctors frequently looked at a computer screen during an examination.

Recent studies have found that physicians actually spend more time on electronic documentation than on providing direct patient care, and other studies have reported that clinical computer work constitutes the highest proportion of time spent by physicians. The breakdown is jarring: Physicians spend an average of 43 percent of their time on data entry and just 28 percent directly caring for patients.

It's easy to ask ourselves if the time required for EMR systems is time well spent. But it's important to keep our perspective. We're still in the initial phases of the digitization of medical records, which means there will be kinks to work out. Over time, as functionality, accessibility, and transparency continue to improve, we'll realize the true potential of this technology. After all, the goal of technology in medicine is to eliminate shadow work for clinicians, to increase standards of care for patients, and to allow doctors to focus on the job we love most—direct patient care.

Contrary to the expected grumbling that accompanies big changes within the medical industry, technology is going to augment, not diminish, the humanistic attributes of medical care.

Here's how this is going to be realized: Currently, most patients' information is manually entered into an electronic health record, typically by a doctor, nurse, or other healthcare staff. Once inbuilt sensors are able to collect data from within the body and machine-to-machine communication occurs without the involvement of human data entry and cognitive labor, the real potential of technology will be realized.

Even as record-keeping is becoming more streamlined, medical decision-making is still best performed by the physicians involved in a particular patient's care. Cognitive aptitude (or inaptitude) of a medical professional is the only method through which treatment choices are proposed to patients.

Eventually, though, the most prized of our unique assets—human cognition—will be supplanted by technology, too. As J.C.R Licklider observed in his seminal 1960 paper, "Man-Computer Symbiosis," "Most of the time devoted to problem-solving done by humans can be done most effectively by machines." He continued:

> If those problems can be solved in such a way as to create a symbiotic relation between a man and a fast information-retrieval and data-processing machine, however, it seems evident that the cooperative interaction would greatly improve the thinking process.

In general, technology will carry out, as Licklider puts it, the "routinizable" operations that fill the intervals between decisions. And as we continue to make forward strides, technology will eventually surpass the routinizable to perform many specialized tasks.

As doctors continue to attempt to keep up with a knowledge base that's expanding exponentially, the natural next step in this evolution of medicine is the digitization of the diagnostic approach—the ability to curb human error and cognitive limitation from the decision-making process. Technology is able to provide support to make timely decisions, further standardize medical practice, and provide more data for research than ever before. Through data analytics, we will be able to sift through mounds of data to gain levels of insight never before possible, thus providing new and improved conclusions to long-existing problems.

The entire patient-physician encounter is being largely computerized, with applications designed to aid clinicians in everything from diagnosing to developing treatment strategies. These applications serve as a sort of care continuum the doctor follows throughout the appointment, providing quick access to data-driven decision-making and the ability to alert the physician to previously unrecognized patterns within a patient's history. The distinct characteristics of individual patients are then analyzed against the computer's massive knowledge base that includes all academic literature, all possibly relevant genetic mutations, and all the clinical trials that target these particular mutations to generate patient-specific recommendations. The system then presents the doctor with reports outlining various options and treatment alternatives, as well as explaining how it came to these conclusions by referencing the original data. Cognitive support to physicians extends to include reminders of overdue preventative measures, advice for prescribing, critiques of existing orders, and suggestions for active care. These decision-support systems are ideally geared to save the clinician time and the patient money.

Technology has far more capacity to consider variables than the average doctor could ever hope to do, all the while leaving much less room for error. A doctor can't remember the last 200 research articles on a specific heart disease, for instance, but a computer can. Technology can provide a multitude of options for patients to choose from, based on real-time data and the latest available research. This influx of health data will change the game forever. Once we have a large enough data set and an addressable database of research studies, we'll be able to identify patterns and physiological interactions in ways never before possible.

At present, many computerized diagnosis aids do not yet measure up to the performance of human doctors. But when this happens, the doctor will be released from a number of cognitive activities that can instead be automated. Future bioprocessors, for instance, will not only gather information, but could also diagnose illnesses and even forecast our health. They'll give us instantaneous analysis of various parameters, including cholesterol levels, stress-hormone levels, tissue perfusion, oxygen-saturation levels, blood pressure, blood sugar, heart rate, body temperature, sleep habits, exercise patterns, eating habits, family history, and genetic sequencing. A risk profile could then be generated using these data points, incorporating the latest research to make predictions about a patient's well-being. And all of this could occur without the active participation of the physician.

A high-tech brain pacemaker that could internally communicate with a continuous blood-glucose monitoring device, for example, might detect that an individual's blood sugar is low. This, in turn, could identify those individuals who might potentially have a seizure when their blood sugar drops to critically low levels. The brain pacemaker would then send feedback messages to the pancreas to temporarily inhibit insulin release and immediately correct these sugar levels to avert the seizure. If a seizure was still imminent, then the pacemaker might instead autocorrect the electrical signals within that part of the brain and prevent the seizure from occurring.

One of the most exciting parts of this entire process is that all of these events could later be retrieved from the recorded data, just like the black box of an airplane. Biometric devices will make internal monitoring systems transparent, allowing us to use the information these systems are gathering to better react to medical emergencies like strokes and heart attacks.

In the near future, technology is going to be able to answer many routine questions that patients ask surgeons before they go under the scalpel: What's the success rate of this procedure? How long is the recovery? How much time should I take off from work? How will this impact the rest of my life? Eventually, technology might provide the answers with *you* in mind instead of just being based on population statistics alone, which is the standard practice today.

As we extend our human abilities with new tools and as nascent artificial intelligence matures and makes its way into our workflows, we'll enter a new period of bioelectronics. We will see medical research grow more and more individualized, a metamorphosis beyond labs or in controlled randomized studies. Through the use of real-time data, 3D visualizations, virtual reality, and lifelike digital simulations, what we'll see is that research and education, as well as practical application of care, can eventually become customized for every patient.

The goal of the digitization of the cognitive process is to circumvent limitations of human decision-making. Technology will help eliminate some of the many errors that naturally occur in our current medical climate. And although technology can help reduce our errors, it can never create a fully error-free system for one simple reason: Machines are built and designed by human agency, and we will unavoidably transfer some element of our own limitations onto them. Regardless of how much technology augments areas of medicine, we will always need an expert to guide a machine through the scope of choices or specifics technology provides. In one capacity or another, human touch is indispensable for the foreseeable future.

Nevertheless, the transformation offered by technology will grant physicians more time and opportunities to be involved in the emotional and existential needs of patients. For doctors who are too preoccupied with a disease-centered approach, this shift will allow practitioners to focus more fully on patient-centered care.

Training in present-day medical schools has already started to incorporate didactics in interpersonal skills to address the existential needs of the sick. Instructors will continue to teach these skills, along with professionalism and other communication tactics, with as much emphasis as is currently placed on the instruction of clinical acumen. The age-old apprenticeship model of learning to diagnose diseases or training in surgical skills from experienced teachers will be largely replaced by simulators.

However, at each major disruption in medical technology, there will be resistance among primary stakeholders—doctors and patients—as they adjust to these new systems. Throughout the nineteenth century, we treated symptoms. In the twentieth century, we treated diseases. In the twenty-first century, technology will increasingly predict and prevent disease—and when it can't, it will replace damaged and failing organs at impressive rates.

In the future, a further separation of medicine into two fields—art and science—is going to become even more visible. Technology will replace the scientific side of a doctor's practice and will allow them to focus instead on a more personalized approach to healing, restoring the art of medicine in the process. It's hard to imagine now, but as our technology becomes more advanced and ubiquitous, we might grow that much more human. Doctors will remain as the face of this science because of the breadth and depth of their day-to-day interactions with the sick and dying. Technology experts, biochemical researchers, and entrepreneurs—while critical players—will remain their collaborators. And it's this collective team of experts working together that will propel us into new frontiers of healthcare.

CHAPTER 18

HOW WE MADE THE MODERN DOCTOR

> What patients seek is not scientific knowledge that doctors hide but existential authenticity each person must find on her own. Getting too deeply into statistics is like trying to quench a thirst with salty water. The angst of facing mortality has no remedy in probability.
>
> —PAUL KALANITHI

Each of us is a collage of the various social, religious, and technological changes we've experienced throughout our lives. In the interaction between physicians and patients, these influences determine how decisions are made and how outcomes are managed.

Regardless of how well science and technology have progressed to solve medical problems, and regardless of how well we've prepared ourselves to care for our emotional needs, we as patients continue to struggle to cope with one main issue.

When we're faced with difficult situations, such as when we or someone we love is suffering from an incurable illness, we sometimes find ourselves caught up in a *why me?* or *why them?* line of thinking. These questions are common, but for medical professionals, they're among the most difficult to answer.

David Steensma writes about this tricky dichotomy he navigates with patients in his book, *The Art of Oncology: When the Tumor Is Not the Target*:

> Why do some people who smoke get lung cancer while other heavy smokers remain healthy? Why do some people who do not smoke at all still develop the disease? A detailed understanding of host susceptibility patterns may clarify molecular murkiness, but can't explain away the seeming injustice.

It's that sense of injustice that drives patients to wonder why they've been handed a particular diagnosis. It's our nature to seek answers and to rationalize random misfortune with sentimental interpretations. These ideas are instilled in us by our culture—perhaps that we suffer because we have sinned, and only through the correct beliefs can we be rid of the suffering. Or that our suffering is the result of past karma, and the only way out of the misery is by doing good deeds. Or that suffering is a path to salvation and ought to be accepted with humility. As the Anglican John Betjeman wrote, "Oh! I bless the good Lord for my Boils. For my mental and bodily pains. For without them my Faith all congeals. And I'm doomed to HELL's NE'ER-ENDING FLAMES."

We rely on this glorified rationalization as a way to explain why we suffer. Obviously, these convictions cannot be scientifically proven—they are not testable hypotheses. However, for those who hold these beliefs, a great deal of existential confusion seems to suddenly make sense. For some believers, this affords satisfactory reasons for the perplexing problems and complicated affairs of human life. It's a tough pill to swallow that our lot in life is random, that sometimes good people just get unlucky, that you can do everything "right" and still that might not be enough. To believe instead that our illnesses are a result of our sins but also that there is everlasting salvation in our future can offer stark relief.

Even for those of us who believe that being pious has nothing to do with being stricken by illness, we often still can't help but ponder within these spaces. We may not be the same people as our ancestors, but some of their beliefs are forever locked into our psyches. We're shaped by the accumulated wisdom, practices, traditions, and cultures of those who lived before us. These familiar beliefs and pervasive practices have left an indelible mark, both in our minds and on our DNA.

Whether or not we seek answers from a culture or religion, many of us do search high and low for a personal confidant in our physician. For certain health problems, there's no manual that gives us the right answer. Sometimes, there simply is no right answer. To embrace uncertainty, we need an understanding, an explanation, and—more than anything—a reassurance of a meaningful life. Those who are terminally ill may yearn for a touch of metaphysics, a narrative that has nothing to do with what science offers. To cope with death, we sometimes need a story that connects us with eternity.

For a patient, medical professionals are a critical line of defense, and this means we may also share a disproportionate burden of responsibility for a patient's outcome. Anatole Broyard, longtime *New York Times* book critic, wrote of his ideal doctor in his book *Intoxicated by My Illness* while dying of prostate cancer:

> I would like a doctor who is not only a talented physician, but a bit of a metaphysician, too. Someone who can treat body and soul. There's a physical self who's ill, and there's a metaphysical self who's ill.

But the relationship Broyard describes almost never occurs in a modern patient-physician encounter. With its technological advances, medical science may track genetic mutations; find ways to edit our genes; and forecast, treat, cure, and prevent diseases from occurring, but there's no provision to answer the sublime questions of those who are suffering.

One inadequacy of modern medical science is that it's perceived by some as unemotional and rigid. But this mechanical approach is the very thing that provided the field of medicine and biology with a set of tools for methodical investigation and for a new, self-assured identity. It took nearly three centuries to systematically eliminate doctrinism from the medical profession. The doctor, by necessity, became a scientist, and the study of medicine in turn became mechanistic. It is *this* culture of medicine that takes the center seat in patient-physician interactions.

The complexity of biology made it necessary for ancient physicians to shift from the polymaths of antiquity to highly specialized experts in the modern era. Great scientific minds worked together to aid doctors in understanding the human body through the use of mathematical models, physical laws, and chemical reactions. Medical scientists elevated their work with the help of physicists, chemists, and mathematicians. The lines between organic and inorganic processes were thus deemed nonexistent.

In this modern era of medicine, each specialist studies the human organism from their own viewpoint. An evolutionary biologist looks at the human body as a receptacle programmed by nature, the sole aim of which is to propagate copies of its genes. A biochemist approaches the human body as a complex network of chemical signaling. A biotechnologist sees it as a playing field where principles of engineering are applied to tissues, cells, and molecules to improve early detection of illnesses, the manufacturing of drugs, and the identification of genetic disease. A biostatistician studies the human organism as a quantitative data field where metrics are extracted and analyzed to provide objective information about bodily functions.

The physician is now challenged with looking at the human body for what it is—a dynamic interplay of many known and unknown variables—while providing care that's individualized with *you* in mind.

. . .

Excessive specialization, a mechanistic outlook, and consumerism (including patients' expectations that they ought to be treated as consumers) were all necessary compromises medical professionals had to make in order for the system to run as it needed to. But this shouldn't give modern physicians permission to undermine the existential crises each patient faces when suffering from an illness.

Ancient healers left many gaps to fill, but to advance our understanding of ourselves doesn't always mean that what existed before must be completely destroyed. As physicians in the modern day, we routinely underinvest in our patients' narratives because of the seemingly impenetrable constraints of the modern medical establishment. Vivid, memorable interactions with patients—even if only in the form of a fleeting conversation—remain a critically important part of their care.

Sometimes patients may be seeking something more than tests, procedures, medications, or referrals to another specialist. Perhaps, in conjunction with these things, they want the opportunity to be heard by a professional. But as physicians who have invested in years of highly specialized training, we're brainwashed into thinking that something tangible—to order a test, perform a surgery, or prescribe a drug—is what we always ought to be doing. For certain patients, simply listening can be a treatment—or at least a key part of it. To go beyond the provision of "standard" medical care to become a patient's trusted advocate provides an immeasurable service.

We all have stories to tell. The emotions, feelings, and actions that make up our individual narratives have effects, directly or indirectly, on our physical and mental health. For each of us, our life story conceals within it the innumerable threads that weave together our mind and body. As we live these stories, a few pervasive habits can wreak havoc on our health. By revisiting an individual's narrative, a physician sometimes has the power to rewrite harmful patterns for a new beginning in a better, happier story.

To harness this ability, a physician must encompass certain attributes of the ancient healer, while at the same time differentiating as a specialized individual who can deal with the enormity of caring for human life. We're tasked with carrying forward the timeless principles of the profession: to cure as often as we can, to relieve when we cannot cure, and, always, to comfort.

Part mathematician, part physicist, part chemist, part technologist, part empathetic listener, part counselor, part patient well-wisher, and part philosopher—each combine to make the modern doctor. Only by exploring this identity of modern physicians, by looking more deeply at the byproducts of the innumerable layers of social, cultural, and technological changes that have shaped us, will we be able to fully recognize the enormity of our role.

TO MY FELLOW AND FUTURE DOCTORS

ON TECHNOLOGY ~

Acknowledge this reality: Technology is always going to affect how you practice medicine. Among all fields of human advancement, medicine will likely see the most changes. Embrace them. If you're not going to be part of the way forward, someone else will be. The worst thing you can do is to banish these new developments or to hide from them. In doing so, you're disenfranchising yourself from the progress and surrendering your autonomy to powers outside of the profession. Instead, take them in stride from the start. The incorporation of newer technologies into medical practice is inevitable—your task is to be part of the revolution and to blossom within it.

Present in every technology, at each stage of its evolution, is not only the potential for greater benefit, but also an equal potential to cause mistakes or to be abused. It's our responsibility to continue to improve man-made systems to serve us better, but we shouldn't forget that technology is filled with both possibility and destruction. Like raising a child or teaching a student, technology must be steered so that its talents are matched correctly to its inherent skills. Technology can bring to fruition the vision of personalized medicine, but it also leaves far too many options from which to choose.

ON SLOWING DOWN ~

Our entire healthcare system, dominated by market forces and routinized practices, has become stuck in the fast lane. It hasn't always been this way, but this is the result of our industrialization mentality, of the perception that "time is money." Doctors are allotted only bite-sized amounts of time, most commonly 10 or 15 minutes, to see each patient. In this brief window, we're expected to evaluate an individual, discuss test results, educate, explain a treatment plan, talk to family members, and fill out relevant paperwork and complete charting. We're also expected to identify and respond to patients' expectations and fears and to check patients' understanding of their diagnoses and recommended alternate treatments.

Much of our training has led us to quickly navigate through these hurdles, simply trying to survive the day. When we rush from patient to patient, it's easy to focus on the illness, seeing someone only as a collection of signs and symptoms. We feel the crunch more than ever, and we pick up habits that we don't necessarily want—such as interrupting patients—as we try to find ways to stay accountable to the clock.

In a world of overpacked schedules and high-pressure performance measures, calling for change becomes important. Slowing down the process of care allows patients to take part in it. It strengthens the relationships between doctors and patients. This is a gain for both parties.

Beyond the obvious benefit of really listening to our patients, slowing down has a broader impact: mindfulness. When we have more time to examine and talk with a patient, more time to consult with other doctors, re-review lab test results, and carefully consider medications and treatments, we're simply able to provide better care. Mindfulness helps prevent over-testing and over-treating, and it also gives us more time to educate our patients about lifestyle changes as part of a holistic treatment plan.

We have a responsibility to do better in finding a delicate balance between two opposing views: the ancient view of the human body as a garden to be tended, and the modern view of the human body as a machine to be fixed. To provide the education, tools, and supportive environment that activate the body's healing response mechanisms requires patience and time. The happy marriage of technology and the human touch will happen only if we prepare for a change and then work hard to make it happen.

Ultimately, be mindful of your own conditioned thinking and practices. We are so habituated to our fast-paced lifestyle that unless we consistently remind ourselves to slow down, we'll easily slip back into racing mode. Try incorporating moments of silence into your day. Make it a habit to spend time regularly reflecting on your experiences. Use what you discover in these moments to guide you toward not only what you can teach others, but also what you can still learn.

ON WORK ~

There's an old adage that claims "If we do what we love, we won't have to work for a single day of our lives."

This is a misconception. No matter how much you love your work, every job entails certain duties that are simply unpleasant and cumbersome—there's no way around it. For physicians, there are two main sources of frustration.

One is administrative duties. Charting patient records and the incessant back and forth with insurance companies just to get approval for certain medications, treatments, or tests are some of the elements that doctors and nurses typically don't enjoy. But this sort of shadow work lurks in the depths of every job. The key is to not get overly distracted or frustrated by these ancillary tasks, nor to let them undermine our primary goal, which is to care, cure, and comfort the sick.

The second challenge for physicians is the delicate act of dealing with an angry, defensive, manipulative, or non-compliant patient. That takes work. The job of a physician is not easy, and we knew this before we embarked on our journey into this profession. But we signed up for this to serve a higher purpose—to be directly involved in the well-being of others and to see our patients get better because of the work we do. This is true *no matter who our patients are.*

The only way to achieve true happiness in this or any other profession is to express yourself through your skills and enthusiasm. You spent thousands of hours toiling to get here, and the payoff is a sense of purpose.

As physicians and as patients, we have many complaints about the system we collectively created. Positive change arises only out of dissatisfaction with the way things are, coupled with an active desire to steer things toward a more satisfying version of what we know. This is how the big shift happens—by small, incremental changes brought forth by each one of us day after day after day.

There are physicians who long for the return of the old days, those who have made peace with the present, and those who embrace the future of medicine. By whatever means necessary, a genuine healer adapts to the demands of the system we made. What ultimately matters is how far physicians are willing to go to ease another person's suffering. If we compromise on this one objective, doctors will quickly become a disposable commodity. This is our litmus test.

ON COMPASSION ~

Though it's critical to embrace technology, don't underestimate the importance of the humanistic dimension in your practice.

In studying any activity or process of an organic lifeform, we see that a billion interacting deterministic factors influence it. Unraveling these factors became an intractable problem for medical professionals to solve. Fortunately, we invented a method to tackle this dilemma.

With the scientific method, we learned how to control the environment in which we study life processes. It is an objective method of validating the utility of a claim, and it worked. Using this approach, we understood more about the human body in a short span—something we couldn't do for millennia. After a while, however, we took the process for granted. We forgot that this approach omits some of the most prized human attributes: our fears, beliefs, and biases when we encounter existential crises.

The scientific method provided us with verifiable knowledge. This is priceless. But living under the false assurance of knowledge, the notion that if something is not measurable, it is not important, is worse than ignorance.

Don't get lost in the convention of "only things that can be measured are the ones I agree to tend." This is blocked thinking. As physicians, we sometimes get lost in the activities with measurable outcomes, focusing all of our attention on the pieces of the puzzle that can be monitored and recorded. Yet many other elements within the way we practice care cannot be quantified but are equally important.

When you encounter a chronic or terminal illness in an individual, it's disingenuous to hide under the false assurance of technology. When you've used up everything that science has to offer, don't be afraid to embrace your own emotional vulnerability. What really matters to a patient when all else fails is the presence of a comforting hand. Whether you do or don't believe in God, or if you believe in a different higher power, it's still okay to acknowledge the patient's faith—a small act of kindness to help someone in a difficult time. Terminal illness is a lonely place. Do all that you can to help your patient navigate this uncharted territory. The full depth of our capacity lies in our compassion.

However much credit we must rightly give to the scientific method, don't let these methods rule your mind. Use them only as guideposts—as tools to help you understand your patients. In the end, each patient is unique. An individual is not a statistic. Even in the age of real-time data analysis, remember that no quantitative analysis can factor in all of the known and unknown contributors affecting someone.

The only solution is a conversation, a deliberate engagement with the person under your care, aided by the use of the correct technology to find the most applicable solutions at the right time. It requires a heart to understand another heart.

Remember that you are not *just* a doctor, you're a doctor-philosopher-educator and many things all in one, each merged by degrees into a single identity. Be generous. Realize that, despite any advances in medicine, no one can cure death. But *you* as a healer have the ability to help cure the fear of death in the person under your care. This, to some patients, means everything.

Notes on Sources

CHAPTER 1—THE NATURAL PHILOSOPHER

1. "research finds that most of the mutations": Tomasetti, C., Li, L., & Vogelstein, B. (2017). Stem cell divisions, somatic mutations, cancer etiology, and cancer prevention. *Science*, 355(6331), 1330-1334. doi:10.1126/science.aaf9011

2. "mutation that occurred about 15 million years ago": Johnson, R. J., Merriman, T., & Lanaspa, M. A. (2015). Causal or Noncausal Relationship of Uric Acid With Diabetes: Table 1. *Diabetes*, 64(8), 2720–2722.

3. "English physician Thomas Sydenham": Sydenham, T., & Wallis, G. (1971). *A treatise of the gout and dropsy*. Philadelphia?: Reprinted with the permission of the Library of the College of Physicians of Philadelphia, 185.

4. "evolutionary explanation of a disease": Nesse, R. M., & Williams, G. C. (1994). *Why we get sick: The new science of Darwinian medicine*. New York: Times Books.

5. "power behind the words": University of Pittsburgh, Schools of the Health Sciences. (2013, May 9). Doctor's Choice of Words May Influence Family's Decision to Permit CPR if Critically Ill Patient's Heart Stops [Press release]. Retrieved from http://www.upmc.com/media/NewsReleases/2013/Pages/doctors-choice-of-words-influence-cpr-decision.aspx

6. "One popular belief of pre-medieval times": Chadwick, N. K. (1936). Shamanism Among the Tatars of Central Asia. *The Journal of the Royal Anthropological Institute of Great Britain and Ireland*, 66, 97–99.

7. "Edwin Smith Papyrus": Scher, C. S. (2014). *Anesthesia for trauma: New evidence and new challenges*, 8.

8. "physicians classified injuries": Stiefel, M., Shaner, A., & Schaefer, S. D. (2006). The Edwin Smith Papyrus: The Birth of Analytical Thinking in Medicine and Otolaryngology. *The Laryngoscope*, 116(2), 182–188.

9. "to comfort always": Knopf, S. A. (1922). *A history of the National tuberculosis association; the anti-tuberculosis movement in the United States*. New York City: National Tuberculosis Association, 320.

10. "must be preserved intact": Waddock, S. A. (2015). *Intellectual shamans: Management academics making a difference*. Cambridge: Cambridge University Press, 138.

11. "soul survives unharmed": Philosophy of Mind – Ancient and Medieval – Ancient Greek And Roman Views. (n.d.). Retrieved March 01, 2015, from http://science .jrank.org/pages/10723/Philosophy-Mind-Ancient-Medieval-Ancient-Greek -Roman-Views.html

12. "his 'first-cause' principle": Ross, W. D. (2004). *Aristotle* (6th ed.). New York: Routledge, 188, 190.

13. "predicated on anything else": Brann, E. T. (1999). *What, then, is time?* Lanham, MD: Rowman & Littlefield, 37.

14. "*psukhe*": Elliott, J., & Attridge, D. (2011). *Theory after 'theory.'* New York: Routledge, 190.

15. "natural philosophers": Cahan, D. (2003). *From natural philosophy to the sciences: Writing the history of nineteenth-century science*. Chicago: University of Chicago Press.

16. "All things in nature need water": Smith, W. (1867). *Dictionary of Greek and Roman biography and mythology*. Boston: Little, Brown, 1016.

17. "alpha and omega of all things": Seife, C. (2003). *Alpha and Omega: The search for the beginning and end of the universe*. New York: Viking.

18. "eye of the god Horus": Stokstad, M. (2007). Chapter 3: Art of Ancient Egypt. In *Art History* (3rd ed., Vol. 1). Upper Saddle River, NJ: Pearson Prentice Hall.

19. "finely tuned musical instrument": Riedweg, C., & Rendall, S. (2005). *Pythagoras: His life, teaching, and influence*. Ithaca: Cornell University Press, Preface, 80.

20. "blood poisoning": Angus, D. C., & Poll, T. V. (2013). Severe Sepsis and Septic Shock. *New England Journal of Medicine*, 369(9), 840–851.

21. "still in use": Marx, J. A., Hockberger, R. S., Walls, R. M., & Adams, J. (2002). *Rosen's emergency medicine: Concepts and clinical practice* (8th ed.). St. Louis: Mosby, Chapter 138.

22. "particular humoral makeup": Humoral Theory. (n.d.). Retrieved February 02, 2016, from http://ocp.hul.harvard.edu/contagion/humoraltheory.html

23. *"dyscrasia"*: Haubrich, W. S. (1997). *Medical meanings: A glossary of word origins* (2nd ed.). Philadelphia, PA: American College of Physicians, 71.

24. "Empedocles": Frazee, C. A. (1997). *World history: Volume 1, ancient and medieval times to A.D. 1500.* Hauppauge, NY: Barron's Educational Series, 169.

25. "man's theory of sickness": Gordon, R. (1993). *The alarming history of medicine: Amusing anecdotes from Hippocrates to heart transplants.* New York: St. Martin's Griffin, 4.

26. "lineage around 460 BC": H., & Adams, F. (1891). *The genuine works of Hippocrates: Translated from the Greek, with a preliminary discourse and annotations.* New York: William Wood, 19.

27. "black bile represented": Sargent, S. S. (1950). *Social psychology, an integrative interpretation.* New York: Ronald Press, 50.

28. "humors were out of balance": Haubrich, W. S. (2003). *Medical meanings: A glossary of word origins* (2nd ed.). Philadelphia, PA: American College of Physicians, 71.

29. "demonic possession and epilepsy": Chaudhary, U. J., Duncan, J. S., & Lemieux, L. (2011). A dialogue with historical concepts of epilepsy from the Babylonians to Hughlings Jackson: Persistent beliefs. *Epilepsy & Behavior*, 21(2), 109–114.

30. "Before the gods": Diehl, C., & Perkins, E. R. (1893). *Excursions in Greece to recently explored sites of classical interest: Mycenae, Tiryns, Dodona, Delos, Athens, Olympia, Eleusis, Epidaurus, Tanagra: A popular account of the results of recent excavations.* London: H. Grevel, 347.

31. "I swear by Apollo": Major, R. H. (1954). *A history of medicine* (Vol. 1). Springfield, IL: Thomas, 120.

32. "only nature's assistant": Wigmore, A. (1984). *The Hippocrates diet and health program.* Wayne, NJ: Avery Pub. Group, 13.

33. "according to his pupils": Major, R. H. (1954). *A history of medicine* (Vol. 1). Springfield, IL: Thomas, 123.

34. "It is impossible to": Major, R. H. (1954). *A history of medicine* (Vol. 1). Springfield, IL: Thomas, 121.

35. "Hippocrates sought to free medicine": Major, R. H. (1954). *A history of medicine* (Vol. 1). Springfield, IL: Thomas, 138.

CHAPTER 2—INTELLECTUAL HIBERNATION

1. "Charaka": Salwi, D.M. *Scientists of India*. Published by Children's Book Trust, 1986.

2. "Rome has but one": Tiner, J. H. (2001). *Exploring the history of medicine: From the ancient physicians of Pharaoh to genetic engineering*. Green Forest, AR: Master Books, 10.

3. "the most brilliant": Mattern, S. P. (2013). *The prince of medicine: Galen in the Roman Empire*. New York, NY: Oxford University Press, 186.

4. "nearly half of all the literature": Ustun, C. (2004). Galen and his anatomic eponym: Vein of Galen. *Clinical Anatomy*, 17(6), 454–457.

5. "60 gladiator deaths": Nutton, V. (1973). The Chronology of Galen's Early Career. *The Classical Quarterly*, 23(01), 158–171.

6. "added the layer of seasons": Brain, P., & G. (1986). *Galen on bloodletting: A study of the origins, development, and validity of his opinions, with a translation of the three works*. Cambridge: Cambridge University Press, 7 and 8.

7. "to spread *pneuma*": Brain, P., & G. (1986). *Galen on bloodletting: A study of the origins, development, and validity of his opinions, with a translation of the three works*. Cambridge: Cambridge University Press.

8. "single unified system": G., Furley, D. J., & Wilkie, J. S. (1984). *Galen on respiration and the arteries*. Princeton, NJ: Princeton University Press.

9. "spirit which is in heaven": Tiner, J. H. (2001). *Exploring the history of medicine: From the ancient physicians of Pharaoh to genetic engineering*. Green Forest, AR: Master Books, 10.

10. "mental or rational": Ancient Theories of Soul. (2004). In *Stanford encyclopedia of philosophy*. Stanford, CA: Stanford University, Metaphysics Research Lab.

11. "Galen strengthened the relationship": Pergameni, C. (1992). Odysseas Hatzopoulos, ed: *That the best physician is also a philosopher*, with a Modern Greek Translation. Athens, Greece: Odysseas Hatzopoulos & Company, Kaktos Editions.

12. "Hippocrates' Art": Brain, P. (1977). Galen on the Ideal of the Physician. *South African Medical Journal*, 937. Retrieved from http://archive.samj.org.za/1977 VOL LI Jul-Dec/Articles/11 November/4.10 HISTORY OF MEDICINE – GALEN ON THE IDEAL OF THE PHYSICIAN. P. Brain.pdf

13. "Rome's collapse": Bury, J. B. (1908). *A history of the Roman Empire: From its foundations to the death of Marcus Aurelius (27 B.C.-180 A.D.)* (Vol. 1). London: J. Murray.

14. "prohibition of public dissection" Cheung, P. (2007). *Public trust in medical research?: Ethics, law and accountability.* Oxford: Radcliffe, 36.

15. "ban on dissection lifted": Wright, T. (2013). *William Harvey: A life in circulation.* Oxford: Oxford University Press, 34.

16. "shall cut off his fingers": *The Medical world* (Vol. 23). (1905). London: Medico-Political Union, 459.

17. "four pillars of medicine": Paracelsus Bio. (n.d.). Retrieved March 08, 2016, from http://www.ediblewildfood.com/bios/paracelsus.aspx

18. "wisdom of the Creator": Major, R. H. (1954). *A history of medicine* (Vol. 1). Springfield, IL: Thomas, 195

19. "disrespectfully of Galen": Wright, T. (2013). *William Harvey: A life in circulation.* Oxford: Oxford University Press, 80.

20. "*Yathrib*": Quran 33:13, Oxford World's Classics edition.

21. "was the first civilization": Al-Khalili, J. (2011). *The house of wisdom: How Arabic science saved ancient knowledge and gave us the Renaissance.* New York: Penguin Press, Chapter 6: Big Science.

22. "first to crack": Haddad, S. I., Khairallah, A. A., Al-Nafis, I., & A. (1936). *A forgotten chapter in the history of the circulation of the blood.* Philadelphia.

23. "Just because a drug is given": Nasser, M., Tibi, A., & Savage-Smith, E. (2009). Ibn Sina's Canon of Medicine: 11th century rules for assessing the effects of drugs. *J R Soc Med*, 102(2), 78–80.

24. "Qur'an by age 10": Khorasani, S., Addin S., *Islamic Great Encyclopedia,* "Solar," 1367.

25. "*physi* literally means *nature*": Ayers, D. M. (1965). *English words from Latin and Greek elements.* Tucson: University of Arizona Press, 182.

26. "three energies": Tiwari, M. (1995). *Ayurveda secrets of healing: The complete Ayurvedic guide to healing through Pancha Karma seasonal therapies, diet, herbal remedies, and memory.* Twin Lakes, WI: Lotus Press, 31.

27. "Pitta was associated": S. (1999). *A treatise on Ayurveda: Pharmaceutics and therapies: Being an English translation of Śārṅgadhara Saṁhita.* Delhi, India: Sri Satguru, 58.

28. "40 percent of Egypt's population": Egypt – Major Cities (http://countrystudies .us/egypt/57.htm), U.S. Library of Congress.

29. "60 percent perish": Snell, M. (n.d.). The Great Mortality. Retrieved April 19, 2009, from http://historymedren.about.com/

30. "third of Europe died": Wade, N. (2010, October 31). Europe's Plagues Came From China, Study Finds. *New York Times*. Retrieved November 1, 2010, from http://www.nytimes.com/2010/11/01/health/01plague.html?_r=0

31. "Susruta": Major, R. H. (1954). *A history of medicine*. Springfield, IL: Thomas, 68.

32. "Zhang Qian": Loewe, M. (2000). *A biographical dictionary of the Qin, former Han and Xin periods, 221 BC – AD 24*. Leiden: Brill.

33. "Emperor Huang Ti": Veith, I. (1966). *Huang Di nei jing su wen: The Yellow Emperor's classic of internal medicine*. Berkeley, CA: University of California Press.

34. "Hua Tuo": Zimmerman, L. M., & Veith, I. (1961). *Great ideas in the history of surgery*. Baltimore: Williams & Wilkins, 69.

35. "*Chi*": Liao, W. (2009). *Chi: Discovering your life energy*. Boston: Shambhala, Ch. 1.

36. "Girolamo Fracastoro": Nutton, V. (1990). The Reception of Fracastoro's Theory of Contagion: The Seed That Fell among Thorns? *Osiris*, 6, 2nd ser., 196–234.

CHAPTER 3—BREAKING THE IRON MOLD

1. "unmarked grave": Gera, V. (2010, May 22). After 467 years, Copernicus gets a hero's burial. Retrieved from http://www.independent.co.uk/news/world/europe/after-467-years-copernicus-gets-a-heros-burial-1980493.html

2. "first printed copy": Copernicus, N. (1972). *On the Revolutions of the Heavenly Bodies*. London: Macmillan, 3–5.

3. "last breath in 1543": Prowe, L. F. (1967). *Nicolaus Copernicus*. Osnabrück: O. Zeller.

4. "*On the Fabric of the Human Body*": Magner, L. N. (1979). *A history of the life sciences*. New York: M. Dekker, 83.

5. "less is offered": Castiglioni, A. (1943). Andreas Vesalius: Professor at the Medical School of Padua. *Bull N Y Acad Med*, 19(11), 766–777. Retrieved from http://www.ncbi.nlm.nih.gov/pubmed/19312345

6. "200 of Galen's errors": Wright, T. (2013). *William Harvey: A life in circulation*. Oxford: Oxford University Press, 38.

7. "tanned human skin": Johnson, M. (2006, January 11). Libraries Have Books Bound in Human Skin. *Associated Press Online*. Retrieved October 6, 2006, from http://www.highbeam.com/doc/1P1-117172580.html?refid=easy_hf

8. "Vesalius looked to the young artist Johann Stephan Van Calcar": Vesalius, A., Richardson, W. F., & Carman, J. B. (1999). *On the fabric of the human body.* San Francisco: Norman Pub.

9. "Johann Stephan van Calcar": Hazard, J. (1996). Jan Stephan Van Calcar, a valuable and unrecognized collaborator of Vesalius. *Hist Sci Med, 30*(4), 471–480.

10. "300 elaborate illustrations": http://web.stanford.edu/class/history13/Readings /vesalius.htm

11. "To avoid running afoul": Bk. VI, Ch. 15, p. 594 (1543 ed.), pp. 1202f. (New Fabrica).

12. "two-legged asses": Castiglioni, A. (1943). Andreas Vesalius: Professor at the Medical School of Padua. *Bull N Y Acad Med*, 19(11), 766–777. Retrieved from http://www.ncbi.nlm.nih.gov/pubmed/19312345

13. "The exposition of anatomy": Wright, T. (2013). *William Harvey: A life in circulation.* Oxford: Oxford University Press, 67.

14. "According to Galen": Wright, T. (2013). *William Harvey: A life in circulation.* Oxford: Oxford University Press, 32, 103.

15. "pious Roman Catholic": Sharratt, M. (1996). *Galileo: Decisive innovator.* Cambridge: Cambridge, University Press.

16. "his father impelled him": Reston, J. (2000). *Galileo: A life.* Washington, D.C.: Beard Books.

17. "swinging pendulum": Asimov, I. (1972). *Asimov's biographical encyclopedia of science and technology; the lives and achievements of 1195 great scientists from ancient times to the present, chronologically arranged.* Garden City, NY: Doubleday.

18. "Aristotelian theory of the sun circling the Earth": Lawson, R. M. (2004). *Science in the ancient world: An encyclopedia.* Santa Barbara, CA: ABC-CLIO, 29–30.

19. "in 1615": Hannam, J. (2011). *The genesis of science: How the Christian Middle Ages launched the scientific revolution.* Washington, DC: Regnery Pub, 329-344.

20. "I wanted people to understand": James, C. (2002, October 29). Television Review: Observing The Stars, Channeling Laughton. *New York Times.* Retrieved from http://www.nytimes.com/2002/10/29/arts/television-review -observing-the-stars-channeling-laughton.html

21. "first European to describe pulmonary circulation": Khan, I. A.; Daya, S. K.; Gowda, R. M. Evolution of the theory of circulation. *International Journal of Cardiology, 98*(3): 519–521.

22. "incorrect teachings of Galen": Michelakis, E. D. (2014). Pulmonary Arterial Hypertension: Yesterday, Today, Tomorrow. *Circulation Research, 115*(1), 109–114.

23. "*The Restoration of Christianity*": Goldstone, L., & Goldstone, N. B. (2002). *Out of the flames: The remarkable story of a fearless scholar, a fatal heresy, and one of the rarest books in the world.* New York: Broadway Books, 71–72.

24. "His firm rejection of the concept of the holy Trinity": Dibb, A. M. (2005). *Servetus, Swedenborg and the nature of God.* Lanham, MD: University Press of America, 93.

25. "upon a pyre of his own books": Parker, T. H. (2006). *John Calvin: A biography.* Oxford: Lion, 150–152.

26. "Gasparo Tagliacozzi": Tilney, N. L. (2003). *Transplant: From myth to reality.* New Haven: Yale University Press, 13–14.

27. "We restore, rebuild": Tagliacozzi, G., Goldwyn, R. M., & Thomas, J. H. (1996). *De curtorum chirurgia per insitionem.* New York: Gryphon Editions.

28. "reflecting telescope": Hall, A. R. (1992). *Isaac Newton, adventurer in thought.* Oxford, UK: Blackwell, 63.

29. "his microscopic studies of lungs": Gribbin, J. R., & Gribbin, J. R. (2006). *History of Western science, 1543–2001.* London: Folio, 155.

30. "first man to see his sperm": Yount, L. (1996). *Antoni van Leeuwenhoek: First to see microscopic life.* Springfield, NJ: Enslow, 10.

31. "God hath appointed": Haussy, C. D. (1995). *English sermons: Mirrors of society.* Toulouse: Presses universitaires du Mirail, 150.

CHAPTER 4—THE WONDROUS MACHINE

No References

CHAPTER 5—PARADIGM SHIFT

1. "My way of discovering": Wright, T. (2013). *William Harvey: A life in circulation.* Oxford: Oxford University Press, 140–141.

2. "All depends on keeping": Bacon, F., & Rawley, W. (1860). *The works of Francis Bacon* (Vol. 8). Boston: Brown and Taggart.

3. "philosophers into whom": Wright, T. (2013). *William Harvey: A life in circulation.* Oxford: Oxford University Press, 51.

4. "Aristotle's Prime Mover": Wood, L. W. (2005). *God and history: The dialectical tension of faith and history in modern thought.* Lexington, KY: Emeth Press, 13.

5. "interpreted as the soul or spirit": Gill, M. L. (1989). *Aristotle on substance: The paradox of unity.* Princeton, NJ: Princeton University Press, 42.

6. "necessary demonstration": Pera, M. (1991). *Scienza e retorica.* Roma: Laterza, 60.

7. "motions of a clock?": Wright, T. (2013). *William Harvey: A life in circulation.* Oxford: Oxford University Press, 206.

8. "My thought": Descartes, R., & Veitch, J. (1901). *The method, meditations and philosophy of Descartes.* New York: Tudor Pub, 275.

9. "*Codex on the Flight of Birds*": Leonardo da Vinci's *Codex on the Flight of Birds.* (n.d.). Retrieved March 10, 2015, from https://airandspace.si.edu/exhibitions/codex/codex.cfm#page-1

10. "heart as a mechanical pump": Gribbin, J. (2003). *The scientists: A history of science told through the lives of its greatest inventors.* New York: Random House, 31.

11. "Divide each difficulty": Descartes, R., Veitch, J., & Descartes, R. (2008). *Discourse on the method and the Meditations.* New York: Cosimo, 21.

12. "began to crumble": Aristotelianism. (2016). In *Encyclopædia Britannica.* Retrieved from http://www.britannica.com/topic/Aristotelianism

13. "Age of Enlightenment": Israel, J. I. (2006). *Enlightenment contested: Philosophy, modernity, and the emancipation of man 1670–1752.* Oxford: Oxford University Press, p. v – viii.

14. "Dare to be wise": Kant, I. (1959). *Foundations of the metaphysics of morals, and what is enlightenment?* New York: Liberal Arts Press, 1.

15. "Alexander Pope": Cody, D. (2000, July). Alexander Pope and Philosophy. Retrieved from http://www.victorianweb.org/previctorian/pope/phil.html

CHAPTER 6—EMERGENCE OF A NEW SENTIMENT

1. "in cabbages and kings": Briller, S. A., & Conn, H. L. (1966). *The myocardial cell: Structure, function, and modification by cardiac drugs: Heart Association of Southeastern Pennsylvania*: 3. international symposium: Ed. by Stanley A. Briller and Hadley L. Conn, jr. Philadelphia, 157.

2. "new science": Syfret, R. (1948). *The origins of the Royal Society.* London, 75.

3. "The Invisible College": Wilkins, John (1885–1990). *Dictionary of National Biography.* London: Smith, Elder & Co.

4. "Boyle attacked": Gribbin, J. R., & Gribbin, J. R. (2006). *History of Western science, 1543–2001.* London: Folio, 151.

5. "According to Boyle": Boyle, R. (1661). *The sceptical chymist*. London: J.M. Dent & Sons, 350.

6. "Influenced by Descartes": Martini, A. (2014). *The Renaissance of Science: The Story of the Atom and Chemistry: The magnificent scientists and their fabulous accomplishments, a fantastic dream and journey into the past, present and future in the world of chemistry*, 484.

7. "set in motion by a creator": Garber, D., & Roux, S. (2013). *The mechanization of natural philosophy*. Dordrecht: Springer Science Business Media, 11.

8. "We may suppose": Boyle, R., & Birch, T. (1772). *The works of the Honourable Robert Boyle. In six volumes*. London: Printed for J. and F. Rivington, 107.

9. "The Royal Society": Syfret, R. (1948). *The origins of the Royal Society*. London, 78.

10. "The Royal Society repeatedly said": Martin, J. (1992). *Francis Bacon, the state and the reform of natural philosophy*. Cambridge: Cambridge University Press.

11. "the impetus of Francis Bacon's": Steel, B. (1930). *Sir Francis Bacon: The first modern mind*. Garden City, NY: Doubleday.

12. "God's sensorium": Popkin, R. H. (1999). *The Columbia history of Western philosophy*. New York: Columbia University Press, 436.

13. "incorrect interpretation of Scripture": Boyle, R. (1690). *Reflections on a Theological Distinction*. Ann Arbor: University Microfilms International.

14. "Giovanni Borelli of Italy proved": Thurston, A.J. (1999) Giovanni Borelli and the study of human movement: an historical review. *ANZJ Surg 69*(4):276–288.

15. "The laws of chemistry and physics": Carrel, A. (1935). *Man, the unknown*. New York: Harper & Brothers, 8.

16. "We have found the secret of life": Watson and Crick discover chemical structure of DNA. (28, February). Retrieved March 12, 2016, from http://www.history.com/this-day-in-history/watson-and-crick-discover-chemical-structure-of-dna

17. "credited with founding": Morgagni, G.B. (1903). Founders of Modern Medicine: Giovanni Battista Morgagni (1682–1771). *Medical Library and History Journal 1*(4): 270–7.

18. "Marie-François Bichat": Simmons, J. (2002). *Doctors and discoveries: Lives that created today's medicine*. Boston: Houghton Mifflin, 58.

19. "He has fulfilled": Lesch, J. E. (1984). *Science and medicine in France: The emergence of experimental physiology, 1790–1855*. Cambridge: Harvard University Press.

20. "saved more lives than": Newsholme, A. (1936). *The last thirty years in public health; recollections and reflections on my official and post-official life*. London: Allen & Unwin, 326.

21. "the Declaration of Independence": Jefferson, T., & Holmes, J. (2002). *Thomas Jefferson: A chronology of his thoughts*. Lanham, MD: Rowman & Littlefield.

22. "the ornament of England": Pointer, J. (1749). *Oxoniensis academia: Or, the antiquities and curiosities of the University of Oxford Giving an account of all the public edifices, both ancient and modern. Together with lists of the founders, public benefactors, governors*. London: Printed for S. Birt, 184.

23. "his 'magic' cure": Cook, T. (1838). *The New Monthly Magazine*, 413.

24. "his epitaph reads": Treasure, G. R., & Dawson, I. (1998). *Who's who in British history: Beginnings to 1901*. London: Fitzroy Dearborn, 359.

25. "doctrine of *transplantatio morborum*": Rothschuh, K. E. (1981). Der Ausklang der wissenschaftlichen Iatromagie. *Ber. Wissenschaftsgesch.*, 4:51–60. Retrieved from: http://onlinelibrary.wiley.com/doi/10.1002/bewi.19810040108/abstract

26. "American psychologist John Bovee Dods": Dods, J. B. (1843). *Six lectures on the philosophy of mesmerism: Delivered in the Marlboro' chapel, January 23–28, 1843*. Boston: W.A. Hall &, printers, 68.

27. "Twenty years ago, I discovered": Dods, J. B. (1843). *Six lectures on the philosophy of mesmerism: Delivered in the Marlboro' chapel, January 23–28, 1843*. Boston: W.A. Hall &, printers, 63.

28. "most puzzling question of the time": Altonen, B., MPH, MS. (2010). Reverend John Bovee Dods. Retrieved from http://brianaltonenmph.com/6-history -of-medicine-and-pharmacy/hudson-valley-medical-history/the-fowler-estate /rev-john-bovee-dods/

29. "Electrical Psychology": Dods, J. B. (1850). *The Philosophy of Electrical Psychology: in a course of twelve lectures, etc.* Fowlers & Wells: New York, 252.

30. "Claude Bernard published": Bernard, C. (1957). *An introduction to the study of experimental medicine*. New York: Dover Publications.

31. "Darwin's Bulldog": Desmond, A. J. (n.d.). Thomas Henry Huxley. Retrieved March 10, 2016, from http://www.britannica.com/biography /Thomas-Henry-Huxley

32. "seven months after its publication": Thomson, K. S. (2000). Huxley, Wilberforce and the Oxford Museum. *American Scientist* 88 (3): 210. doi:10.1511/2000.3.210.

33. "great gifts": Lucas, J. R. (1979). Wilberforce and Huxley: a legendary encounter. *The Historical Journal* 22 (2): 313–330. doi:10.1017/S0018246X00016848. PMID 11617072.

34. "Cyrill Franz Napp , the abbot": Gribbin, J. R. (2006). *History of Western science, 1543–2001*. London: Folio, 583

35. "was introduced to Napp": Hasan, H. (2004). *Mendel and The Laws Of Genetics*. The Rosen Publishing Group. ISBN 9781404203099.

36. "name was changed to Gregor": Henig, R. M. (2000). *The monk in the garden: The lost and found genius of Gregor Mendel, the Father of Genetics*. Boston: Houghton Mifflin, 24.

37. "to obtain a free education": Henig, R. M. (2000). *The Monk in the Garden: The Lost and Found Genius of Gregor Mendel, the Father of Genetics*. Boston: Houghton Mifflin. ISBN 978-0-395-97765-1. 19–21.

38. "duties as the monastic head": Windle, B.C.A. (1911). Mendel, Mendelism. *Catholic Encyclopedia*. Looby, John (trans.). Retrieved 2 April 2007.

39. "rediscovery of Mendel's laws": Bowler, P. J. (2003). *Evolution: the history of an idea*. Berkeley: University of California Press. ISBN 0-520-23693-9.

CHAPTER 7—STUDIES, STUDIES, AND MORE STUDIES

1. "The announcement yesterday"; "I'm just letting all my calls": Kolata, G., & Petersen, M. (2002, July 10). Hormone Replacement Study A Shock to the Medical System. Retrieved December 26, 2016, from http://www.nytimes.com/2002/07/10/us/hormone-replacement-study-a-shock-to-the-medical-system.html

2. "risk of breast cancer": Risks and Benefits of Estrogen Plus Progestin in Healthy Postmenopausal Women: Principal Results From the Women's Health Initiative Randomized Controlled Trial. (2002). *Obstetrical & Gynecological Survey*, 57(11), 750–752.

3. "160,000 women": Parker-Pope, T. (2011). The Women's Health Initiative and the Body Politic. Retrieved December 26, 2016, from http://www.nytimes.com/2011/04/10/weekinreview/10estrogen.html

4. "26 percent increased chance": Findings from the WHI Postmenopausal Hormone Therapy Trials. (2010, September 21). Retrieved December 26, 2016, from http://www.nhlbi.nih.gov/whi/

5. "about 20 percent of menopausal women": Parry, B., MD. (2013). Special Issues in Menopause and Major Depressive Disorder. *Psychiatric Times*. Retrieved December 26, 2016, from http://www.psychiatrictimes.com/bipolar-disorder/special-issues-menopause-and-major-depressive-disorder

6. "a very lively and bubbly woman": Menopause misery drove wife to suicide. (2003). Retrieved December 26, 2016, from http://www.dailymail.co.uk/health/article-189060/Menopause-misery-drove-wife-suicide.html#ixzz4Hmvx6eOY

7. "A storm of 13,000 women": Singer, N. (2009). Menopause, as Brought to You by Big Pharma. Retrieved December 24, 2016, from http://nyti.ms/1U2ktml

8. "Prempro's sales plummeted": Petersen, M. (2002). Wyeth Stock Falls 24% after Report. Retrieved December 24, 2016, from http://www.nytimes.com/2002/07/10/us/wyeth-stock-falls-24-after-report.html

9. "By June 2012": Pfizer Paid $896 Million in Prempro Settlements. (2012). Retrieved December 24, 2016, from http://www.bloomberg.com/news/articles/2012-06-19/pfizer-paid-896-million-in-prempro-accords-filing-shows-1-

10. "saga doesn't end there": Shute, N. (2013, October 4). The Last Word On Hormone Therapy From the Women's Health Initiative. Retrieved December 26, 2016, from http://www.npr.org/sections/health-shots/2013/10/04/229171477/the-last-word-on-hormone-therapy-from-the-womens-health-initiative

11. "conflicting results": Confused about estrogen therapy? (2013, July 19). Retrieved December 26, 2016, from http://thechart.blogs.cnn.com/2013/07/19/confused-about-estrogen-therapy/

12. "there is no clear consensus": Alvarez, D. M. (2006, May 16). Confusion over Hormone Replacement Therapy. Retrieved December 26, 2016, from http://www.foxnews.com/story/2006/05/16/confusion-over-hormone-replacement-therapy.html

CHAPTER 8—HOW MATHEMATICIANS CHANGED MEDICAL PRACTICE

1. "to reject every empirical process": http://www-groups.dcs.st-and.ac.uk/history/Extras/Laplace_mechanique_celeste.html

2. "British physician, Richard Lower": Davis, R. B. (2000). Richard Lower: Anatomist and Physiologist. *Annals of Internal Medicine*, 132(12), 1008.

3. "That this red color": Gribbin, J. R. (2006). *History of Western science, 1543–2001*. London: Folio, 156, 157.

4. "despite his total opposition": Westfall, R. S. (1980). *Never at Rest*. Cambridge University Press, 330–1.

5. "Newton also did not believe": Westfall, R. S. (1980). *Never at Rest*. Cambridge University Press, 315.

6. "Greek philosophers who incorporated": Westfall, R. S. (1980). *Never at Rest*. Cambridge University Press, 315.

7. "Fluxion": Newton, I., Whiteside, D. T., & Hoskin, M. (1967). *The mathematical papers of Isaac Newton* (Vol. 1). Cambridge: Cambridge University Press. In reprint 2008. "The October 1666 Tract on Fluxions," 7:400.

8. "known as calculus": Newton, I. (n.d.). Newton Papers : Newton's Waste Book. Retrieved March 10, 2016, from http://cudl.lib.cam.ac.uk/view/MS-ADD-04004/1 From the Portsmouth Collection, donated by the fifth Earl of Portsmouth, 1872.

9. "Gottfried Leibniz, also developed calculus": Niccolò Guicciardini, (2003). *Reading the Principia: The Debate on Newton's Mathematical Methods for Natural Philosophy from 1687 to 1736*. Cambridge University Press, 250.

10. "John Graunt." Encyclopedia of World Biography. 2004. Retrieved March 10, 2016, from Encyclopedia.com: http://www.encyclopedia.com/doc/1G2-3404707807.html

11. "*Observations*": Graunt, J., & Petty, W. (1665). *Natural and political observations mentioned in a following index, and made upon the bills of mortality*. Oxford: Printed by William Hall for John Martyn, and James Allestry.

12. "in the year 1625 alone": John Graunt Facts. (n.d.). Retrieved March 11, 2016, from http://biography.yourdictionary.com/john-graunt

13. "*Observations* attempted to create": London Bill of Mortality, 1-8 February 1675.

14. "applied to the entire system of human knowledge": Lu, Y., & Fang, J. (2003). *Advanced medical statistics*. New Jersey: World Scientific, 3.

15. "Pierre-Jean-Georges Cabanis attempted to": Lu, Y., & Fang, J. (2003). *Advanced medical statistics*. New Jersey: World Scientific, 4.

16. "Louis believed that": Louis, P. C. A. (1836). *Pathological Researchers on Phthisis*, trans. Charles Cowan. Hilliard, Gray, Boston.

17. "Mesmer was a German physician": Principe, L. (2013). *The secrets of alchemy*. University of Chicago Press, 96.

18. "he termed animal magnetism": Fara. P (1995). An Attractive Theory – Animal Magnetism in Eighteenth-Century England, *History of Science*, 33: 127–77.

19. "France's King Louis XVI appointed Benjamin Franklin": Best, M. A., Neuhauser, D., & Slavin, L. (2003). *Benjamin Franklin: Verification & validation of the scientific process in healthcare as demonstrated by the report of the Royal Commission on Animal Magnetism & Mesmerism*. Victoria, B.C.: Trafford, 7–10.

20. "Joseph Victor Broussais claimed that": Lu, Y., & Fang, J. (2003). *Advanced medical statistics*. New Jersey: World Scientific, 5.

21. "in 1825, France exported 10 million leeches": Gordon, R. (1993). *The alarming history of medicine: amusing anecdotes from Hippocrates to heart transplants*. New York: St. Martin's Griffin, 170.

22. "Among 52 fatal cases": Louis, P. C. A. (1836). (Vols. 1 and 2). translator. Bowditch. H., Butts. I. *Anatomical, Pathological and Therapeutic Researches upon the Disease Known under the Name of Gastro-Enterite Putrid, Adynamic, Ataxix, or Typhoid Fever, etc., Compared with the Most Common Acute Diseases*. Boston.

23. "death rate of the old procedure": Matthews, J. R. (1995). *Quantification and the Quest for Medical Certainty*, Princeton University Press, Princeton, New Jersey.

24. "to establish a commission": Lu, Y., & Fang, J. (2003). *Advanced medical statistics*. New Jersey: World Scientific, 5.

25. "human spirit to the statistical certainty": Double, F. J. (1835). Statistique appliquee a la medicine. *Comptes rendus de l' Académie des Sciences,* 1:281.

26. "a shoemaker who": Lu, Y., & Fang, J. (2003). *Advanced medical statistics*. New Jersey: World Scientific, 6.

27. "Semmelweis's observations were rejected": Carter, K. C., & Carter, B. R. (2005). *Childbed fever: A scientific biography of Ignaz Semmelweis, with a new introduction by the authors*. New Brunswick, NJ: Transaction.

28. "46 percent": Lu, Y., & Fang, J. (2003). *Advanced medical statistics*. New Jersey: World Scientific, 7.

29. "from 1867–70 fell to 15 percent": Lu, Y., & Fang, J. (2003). *Advanced medical statistics*. New Jersey: World Scientific, 7.

30. "Lister published these": Lister, J. (1870). Effects of the antiseptic system of treatment upon the salubrity of a surgical hospital, *The Lancet* i: 40.

31. "plants, animals, and men": Pearson, K. (1911). *The Grammar of Science* (3rd ed.). New York: Macmillan.

32. "medical community began to agree": Kilgore, E. (1920). Relation of Quantitative Methods to the Advance of Medical Science. *Journal of the American Medical Association,* 75(2), 86.

33. "Austin Bradford Hill": Himsworth, Sir Harold. (1982). Bradford Hill and Statistics in Medicine, *Statistics* in Medicine 1:301–302.

34. "The study proved": MRC. (1948). Streptomycin treatment of pulmonary tuberculosis: A Medical Research Council Investigation, *Br. Med. J* 769.

35. "before I tried to get them to run": Hill, A.B. Memories of the British Streptomycin Trial in Tuberculosis – The First Randomized Clinical Trial. *Controlled Clinical Trials* 1990; 11:77–9.

36. "He was a firm believer that": Lu, Y., & Fang, J. (2003). *Advanced medical statistics*. New Jersey: World Scientific, 13.

37. "In 1954, a study was performed": Francis, T. Jr. et al. (1995). An evaluation of the 1954 poliomyelitis vaccines trials – Summary Report, *American Journal of Public Health* 45(5): 1–63.

38. "the largest and most expensive study": Lu, Y., & Fang, J. (2003). *Advanced medical statistics*. New Jersey: World Scientific, 14.

39. "Microbiologists, for instance": Speedy Publishing. (2014). *Calculus Equations And Answers*. Dot EDU. Amazon Digital Services LLC.

40. "Another field that relies on": Kermack, W. O.; McKendrick, A. G. (1927). A Contribution to the Mathematical Theory of Epidemics. *Proceedings of the Royal Society A: Mathematical, Physical and Engineering Sciences*, 115 (772): 700.

41. "helping us mitigate the flu": CDC. (September 26, 2014). Morbidity and Mortality Weekly Report (MMWR). *Updated Preparedness and Response Framework for Influenza Pandemics: Recommendations and Reports.* 63(RR06);1–9.

CHAPTER 9—THE OBSESSION WITH MEASURING THE HUMAN BODY

1. "pendulum clock, invented in 1656": Matthews, M. R. (2000). *Time for science education: how teaching the history and philosophy of pendulum motion can contribute to science literacy*. New York: Springer, 124–126.

2. "Carl Wunderlich conducted a study": Pearce, J. (2002). A brief history of the clinical thermometer. QJM, 95(4), 251–252. Retrieved from http://qjmed .oxfordjournals.org/content/95/4/251

3. "use of the mercury manometer": Booth, J. (1977). A short history of blood pressure measurement. *Proceedings of the Royal Society of Medicine*, 70(11), 793–799.

4. "If I were to call man ape": Gribbin, J. R. (2006). *History of Western science, 1543–2001*. London: Folio, 239.

5. "God's handiwork": Gribbin, J. R. (2006). *History of Western science, 1543–2001.* London: Folio, 240.

6. "Boole had a mystical vision": History of Computers and Computing, Birth of the modern computer, The thinkers, George Boole. (n.d.). Retrieved March 10, 2016, from http://history-computer.com/ModernComputer/thinkers/Boole.html

7. "to unfold the secret laws": Boole, G. (1854). *Investigation of the Laws of Thought on Which are Founded the Mathematical Theories of Logic and Probability.* New York: Dover Publications.

8. "a more deliberate process of observation": Long, L., Jr. (2013, June 1). THE HISTORY OF EXPERIMENTAL PSYCHOLOGY. Retrieved March 10, 2016, from http://psychsocialissues.com/2013/06/01/ the-history-of-experimental-psychology/

9. "love hormones were nothing more than": The chemistry of love: Valentine's Day science from ACS Reactions. (2014, February 10). American Chemical Society. Retrieved March 10, 2016, from http://www.eurekalert.org/pub_ releases/2014-02/acs-tco021014.php

10. "map the areas responsible for love": I want to know where love is – Concordia research helps develop first brain map of love and desire. (2012, June 20). Retrieved March 10, 2016, from http://www.eurekalert.org/pub_releases /2012-06/cu-iwt061912.php

11. "love's scientific basis": Falling in love 'more scientific than you think,' according to Syracuse University professor. (2010, October 22). Retrieved March 10, 2016, from http://www.eurekalert.org/pub_releases/2010-10/su-fil102210.php

12. "All deductions from metaphors": Wright, T. (2013). *William Harvey: A life in circulation.* Oxford: Oxford University Press, 217.

13. "Pythagoras, the forefather of humoral theory": Finger, S. (1994). *Origins of neuroscience: A history of explorations into brain function.* New York: Oxford University Press, 13.

CHAPTER 10—HOW THE HEART LOST ITS ESTEEMED POSITION

1. "we are powerless against": Ornato, J. P., & Peberdy, M. A. (2005). *Cardiopulmonary resuscitation.* Totowa, NJ: Humana Press, 1:3.

2. "When Sherwin Nuland": Gellene, D. (2014). Sherwin B. Nuland, Author of 'How We Die,' Is Dead at 83. Retrieved March 10, 2016, from http://www .nytimes.com/2014/03/05/us/sherwin-b-nuland-author-who-challenged -concept-of-dignified-death-dies-at-83.html?_r=0

3. "open-chest compressions": Nuland, S. B. (1994). *How we die: Reflections on life's final chapter*. New York: A.A. Knopf, 6.

4. "200-pound gadget": W. B. Kouwenhoven, G. G. Knickerbocker. (April 1962). The Development of a Portable Defibrillator. *Transactions of the American Institute of Electrical Engineers. Part III: Power Apparatus and Systems*, 81: 428–431.

5. "heart moves the soul": Webb, H. M. (2004). *The medieval heart: The physiology, poetics and theology of the heart in thirteenth and fourteenth-century Italy*, Yale University Press (March 23, 2010), 26.

6. "Sacred Heart of Jesus": Murphy, J. F. (1951). *Mary's Immaculate Heart; the meaning of the devotion to the Immaculate Heart of Mary*. Milwaukee: Bruce.

7. "feels all, knows all": Wright, T. (2013). *William Harvey: A life in circulation*. Oxford: Oxford University Press, 58.

8. "heart was capable of": Kim, Y. (2000). *The natural philosophy of Chu Hsi (1130–1200)*. Philadelphia: American Philosophical Society, 213.

9. "quixotic ideas to pervade": Wright, T. (2013). *William Harvey: A life in circulation*. Oxford: Oxford University Press, 59.

10. "stage where the emotional action": Shakespeare, W. (1870). *The works of William Shakespeare*. Lennox Collection, 42.

11. "electric fluid": Lewin, W. H., & Goldstein, W. (2011). *For the love of physics: From the end of the rainbow to the edge of time—a journey through the wonders of physics*. New York: Free Press, 128.

12. "Peter Abildgaard announced"; "parties of pleasure": Raising The Dead. (2013, August 25). Retrieved March 10, 2016, from http://drvitelli.typepad.com /providentia/2013/08/the-man-who-raised-the-dead.html

13. "concept of bio-electricity": Whittaker, E. T. (1951). *A history of the theories of aether and electricity*. London: T. Nelson.

14. "Mary Shelley's famous *Frankenstein*": Luigi Galvani. (n.d.). Retrieved March 10, 2016, from http://ethw.org/Luigi_Galvani

15. "argued in papers published in 1792": Kipnis, N. (1987). Luigi Galvani and the debate on animal electricity, 1791–1800. *Annals of Science*, 44(2), 107–142.

16. "came from an outside source": Bresadola, Marco (15 July 1998). Medicine and science in the life of Luigi Galvani. *Brain Research Bulletin* 46 (5): 367–380. doi:10.1016/s0361-9230(98)00023-9.

17. "nerve-conduction experiments": Cajavilca, C., Varon, J., & Sternbach, G. L. (2009). Luigi Galvani and the foundations of electrophysiology. *Resuscitation*, 80(2), 159–162.

18. "15-year-old Hanna Greener": Ferrari, L. R. (1999). *Anesthesia and pain management for the pediatrician*. Baltimore: Johns Hopkins University Press, 30.

19. "the first surgery using": Long, C.W. (1849). An account of the first use of Sulphuric Ether by Inhalation as an Anaesthetic in Surgical Operations. *Southern Medical and Surgical Journal*, 5: 705–13. Retrieved 2010-09-13.

20. "was the first to suggest": Jay, M. (8 August 2014). "O, Excellent Air Bag": Humphry Davy and Nitrous Oxide. *The Public Domain Review* (Open Knowledge Foundation).

21. "Queen Victoria gave birth": Ramsay, M. A. E. (2006). John Snow, MD: anaesthetist to the Queen of England and pioneer epidemiologist. *Proceedings (Baylor University. Medical Center)*, 19(1), 24–28.

22. "Chloroform is a decoy of Satan's": Anonymous. (2012). *The Practitioner*, Volume 60. Ulan Press, 461.

23. "the cries of women": Currie, D., & Raoul, V. (1992). *The Anatomy of gender: Women's struggle for the body*. Ottawa: Carleton University Press, 47.

24. "Greener's accidental death": Snow, J. (1847). *On the inhalation of the vapour of ether in surgical operations: Containing a description of the various stages of etherization, and a statement of the result of nearly eighty operations in which ether has been employed in St. George's and University College Hospitals. London.*

25. "chloroform-induced cardiac arrest": Snow J. (1849). On the fatal cases of the inhalation of chloroform. *Edinburgh Med Surg J*, 72: 75–87.

26. "Ether's staying power": Hake TG. (1874). Studies on ether and chloroform from Professor Schiff's physiological laboratory. *Practitioner*, 12: 241.

27. "after Dr. John McWilliam diligently": McWilliam, J. A. (1889). Electrical Stimulation of the Heart in Man. *British Medical Journal*, 1(1468), 348–350.

28. "by jolting it back": Safar P. (1989). History of cardiopulmonary cerebral resuscitation. In: Kaye W, Bircher N, eds. *Cardiopulmonary Resuscitation*. New York, NY: Churchill Livingstone; 1989: 1–53.

29. "is called *defibrillation*": Prevost J.L, Battelli F. (1899). La mort par les courants electriques-courants alternatifs a haute tension. *J Physiol Pathol*, 1: 427.

30. "While working on dogs": Hooker D.R., Kouwenhoven W.B., Langworthy O.R. (1933). The effect of alternating electrical currents on the heart. *Am J Physiol*, 103: 444–454.

31. "pipe-smoking German professor": Kouwenhoven W.B., Jude J.R., Knickerbocker G.G.(1960). Closed-chest cardiac massage, *JAMA*, 173:94-97.

32. "We didn't have to open her chest": Kouwehhoven, W., & Knickerbocker, G. (1962, october). The Development of a Portable Defibrillator. 428-430. Retrieved from http://em.pgpic.com/docs/ Developmentofaportabledefibrillator(2)_1962_JHU.pdf

33. "This was the breakthrough": Beaudouin, D. (2002, Fall). Reviving the Body Electric: Acclaimed as the "father of cardiopulminary resuscitation" (CPR), William B. Kouwenhoven devoted 50 years to inventing the procedures and devices to jolt a human heart back to life. Johns Hopkins Engineer, 27–32.

34. "CPR was introduced to physicians": History of CPR. (n.d.). Retrieved March 10, 2016, from http://cpr.heart.org/AHAECC/CPRAndECC /AboutCPRFirstAid/HistoryofCPR/UCM_475751_History-of-CPR.jsp

CHAPTER 11—THE UTOPIA OF CURING DEATH

1. "the top end of her thigh bone": Hip Fractures-OrthoInfo – AAOS. (n.d.). Retrieved March 09, 2016, from http://orthoinfo.aaos.org/topic.cfm?topic=A00392

2. "categorized as a hospital-dependent patient": Reuben, D. B., & Tinetti, M. E. (2014). The Hospital-Dependent Patient. *New England Journal of Medicine*, 370(8), 694–697.

3. "92 percent of patients over age 62 obtained": Schonwetter, R. S., Teasdale, T. A., Taffet, G., Robinson, B. E., & Luchi, R. J. (1991). Educating the Elderly: Cardiopulmonary Resuscitation Decisions before and after Intervention. *Journal of the American Geriatrics Society*, 39(4), 372–377.

4. "In a related study, 70 percent of patients": Swor, R. A., Jackson, R. E., Tintinalli, J. E. and Pirrallo, R. G. (2000), Does Advanced Age Matter in Outcomes after Out-of-hospital Cardiac Arrest in Community-dwelling Adults ?. *Academic Emergency Medicine*, 7: 762–768. doi: 10.1111/j.1553-2712.2000.tb02266.x

5. "Dr. Susan Diem and her team": Diem, S., Lantos, J., & Tulsky, J. (1996). Cardiopulmonary resuscitation on television: Miracles and misinformation. *Resuscitation*, 33(1), 96.

6. "On all three shows combined": Adams, D., & Snedden, D. (n.d.). How Misconceptions Among Elderly Patients Regarding Survival Outcomes of Inpatient Cardiopulmonary Resuscitation Affect Do-Not-Resuscitate Orders. Retrieved March 09, 2016, from http://jaoa.org/article.aspx?articleid=2093313

7. "In another study published in August 2015": Portanova, J., Irvine, K., Yi, J. Y., & Enguidanos, S. (2015). It isn't like this on TV: Revisiting CPR survival rates depicted on popular TV shows. *Resuscitation*, 96, 148–150.

8. "7 out of 10 of us say we'd prefer": How We Die. (n.d.). Retrieved March 09, 2016, from http://www.pbs.org/wgbh/pages/frontline/facing-death/facts-and-figures/

9. "to die at home": Cloud, J. (2000). A Kinder, Gentler Death. Retrieved March 09, 2016, from http://content.time.com/time/magazine/article /0,9171,997968,00.html

10. "(more than 70 percent) die in a hospital": NCHS birth and death tables. (2008, October 4). Retrieved March 9, 2016, from http://www.cdc.gov/nchs /data/dvs/Mortfinal2005_worktable_309.pdf

11. "Arab and Jewish doctors": Ofek, H. (2011, Winter). Why the Arabic World Turned Away from Science. Retrieved March 09, 2016, from http://www.thenewatlantis .com/publications/why-the-arabic-world-turned-away-from-science

12. "With all meekness and a calm cheerfulness": Aurelius, M., & Casaubon, M. (1635). *Marcvs Avrelivs Antoninus the Roman Emperovr, his meditations concerning himselfe: Treating of a natvrall mans happinesse ; wherein it consisteth, and of the meanes to attaine unto it.* London: Printed by M. Flesher, for Richard Mynne, 20.

13. "Roman statesman Cicero admired"; "not something to try to outrun": Cicero, M. T., & Bennett, C. E. (1951). *Selections from Cicero: Orations, Letters, and De Senectute.* Boston: Allyn and Bacon, 130, 154.

14. "if we can preserve a dead body by embalming": H, J. (1671). *A treatise of the great antidote of Van Helmont, Paracelsus and Crollius.* London: Publisher not identified.

15. "So great a work as the stopping": Bacon, F., & Rawley, W. (1638). *History naturall and experimentall, of life and death. Or, Of the prolongation of life. Written in Latine.* London: Printed by John Haviland for William Lee, and Humphrey Mosley.

16. "Roger Bacon wrote a treatise on longevity": Haycock, D. B. (2008). *Mortal coil: A short history of living longer.* New Haven: Yale University Press, 21.

17. "we shall have a universal medicine": Haycock, D. B. (2008). *Mortal coil: A short history of living longer.* New Haven: Yale University Press. Chymical, Medicinal and Chyrugical Addresses – Appendix to Eleventh Chapter, 61.

18. "the power of man over matter": Franklin, B., & Franklin, W. T. (1817). *The private correspondence of Benjamin Franklin, LL. D ... comprising a series of letters on miscellaneous, literary, and political subjects.* London: H. Colburn, 52.

19. "disease will be extirpated": Reade, W. W. (1876). *The martyrdom of man*. New York: C.P. Somerby, 514.

20. "kidney dialysis is already routine": Kaufman, S. R., Shim, J. K., & Russ, A. J. (2006). Old Age, Life Extension, and the Character of Medical Choice. *The Journals of Gerontology. Series B, Psychological Sciences and Social Sciences*, 61(4), S175–S184.

21. "has risen by about three months per year": Easterbrook, G. (2014, October). What Happens When We All Live to 100? Retrieved March 09, 2016, from http://www.theatlantic.com/magazine/archive/2014/10/what-happens -when-we-all-live-to-100/379338/

22. "increase 350 percent between 2010 and 2050": Living Longer. (2011, October). Retrieved March 09, 2016, from https://www.nia.nih.gov/research/publication/ global-health-and-aging/living-longer

23. "We live but to create": Comfort, A. (1956). *The biology of senescence*. New York: Rinehart, 5.

24. "the preferred form of death"; "the principle object of mankind": Haycock, D. B. (2008). *Mortal coil: A short history of living longer*. New Haven: Yale University Press, 201, 106.

CHAPTER 12—HOW DOCTORS LOST THE NARRATIVE

1. "we literally share the suffering": Sethi, M. L. (2013, Spring). Are Physicians Wired for Empathy? Retrieved March 9, 2016, from http://archive.protomag.com /assets/are-physicians-wired-for-empathy

2. "experiencing the pain ourselves": Sawamoto, N. et al. (2000, October 1). Expectation of pain enhances responses to nonpainful somatosensory stimulation in the anterior cingulate cortex and parietal operculum/posterior insula: An event-related functional magnetic resonance imaging study. Retrieved March 09, 2016, from http://www.ncbi.nlm.nih.gov/pubmed/11007903

3. "own bodies to produce more stress hormones": Engert, V., Plessow, F., Miller, R., Kirschbaum, C., & Singer, T. (2014, April 30). Your stress is my stress – Merely observing stressful situations can trigger a physical stress response. Retrieved March 09, 2016, from http://www.eurekalert.org/pub_releases/2014-04 /m-ysi043014.php

4. "Listen to your patient": Swartz, M. H. (2014). *Textbook of physical diagnosis: History and examination*. Philadelphia, PA: Saunders/Elsevier, 4.

5. "in his 1912 essay 'Aequanimitas'": Osler, W. (1904). *Aequanimitas, with other addresses to medical students, nurses and practioners of medicine.* London: H.K. Lewis, 6.

6. "see into": Osler, W., & Nelson, J. (1963). *Aequanimitas and other papers that have stood the test of time.* New York: Norton, 29.

7. "These wretched creatures": Wright, T. (2013). *William Harvey: A life in circulation.* Oxford: Oxford University Press, 49.

8. "empathy wanes by the third year of medical school": Sethi, M. L. (2013, Spring). The Need for Compassion. Retrieved March 9, 2016, from http://archive .protomag.com/assets/need-for-compassion?page=1

9. "Event Related Potentials": Decety, J., Yang, C., & Cheng, Y. (2010). Physicians down-regulate their pain empathy response: An event-related brain potential study. *NeuroImage,* 50(4), 1676–1682. Retrieved March 9, 2016.

10. "lamenting the possible failure": Gordon, R. (1994). *The alarming history of medicine.* New York: St. Martin's Press, 129.

11. ""detached concern": Fox R, Lief H. Training for "detached concern." In: Lief, H. (1963). *The Psychological Basis of Medical Practice.* New York, NY: Harper & Row.

12. "Lipps borrowed the word *Einfuhlung*": Coplan, A., & Goldie, P. (2011). *Empathy: Philosophical and psychological perspectives.* Oxford: Oxford University Press.

13. "meaning of empathy was redefined": Halpern, J. (2003). What is clinical empathy? *Journal of General Internal Medicine,* 18(8), 670–674. Retrieved March 9, 2016.

14. "When the Hippocratic *corpus*": Bulger, R. J. (1987). *In search of the modern Hippocrates.* Iowa City: University of Iowa Press, 36.

15. "bad one": French, R. K. (2003). *Medicine before science: the Rational and Learned Doctor from the Middle Ages to the Enlightenment.* New York: Cambridge University Press, 11.

16. "Cicely Saunders completed nursing school at": Dame Cicely Saunders – St Christopher's. (n.d.). Retrieved March 9, 2016, from http://www.stchristophers.org .uk/about/damecicelysaunders

17. "to bring hope and consolation to the end": Saunders, C. M. (2006). *Cicely Saunders: Selected writings 1958–2004.* Oxford: Oxford University Press, 11

18. "she founded the hospice movement in 1967": Richmond, C. (2005). Dame Cicely Saunders. *BMJ : British Medical Journal,* 331(7510), 238.

19. "total pain": Saunders, C. (1963). Management of Intractable Pain. *Proceedings of the Royal Society of Medicine*, 56(3), 195–197.

20. "1.6 million individuals received hospice care": Facts on Hospice and Palliative Care. (n.d.). Retrieved March 09, 2016, from http://www.nhpco.org/hospice -statistics-research-press-room/facts-hospice-and-palliative-care

CHAPTER 13—PRICE TAGS

1. "we may have great and imposing buildings": Dock, L. L., & Stewart, I. M. (1920). *A short history of nursing from the earliest times to the present day*. New York: Putnam, 369.

2. "Who so powerful a fellow laborer": Livingston, R. H. (1981). They comfort me. The history of nursing in Belfast. *The Ulster Medical Journal*, 50(1), 33–45.

3. "hospitium": Buklijaš, T. (2008). Medicine and Society in the Medieval Hospital. *Croatian Medical Journal*, 49(2), 151–154. http://doi.org/10.3325/cmj .2008.2.151

4. "for these sick brethren": Geary, P. J. (2010). *Readings in medieval history*. Toronto: University of Toronto Press, 175.

5. "the Black Death in 1348": Buklijaš, T., & Benyovsky I. (2004). *Domus Christi* in late medieval Dubrovnik: A therapy for the body and soul. *Dubrovnik Annals*, 8:81–107.

6. "Born in Italy": Gill, G. (2005). *The extraordinary upbringing and curious life of Miss Florence Nightingale*. New York: Random House.

7. "Nightingale bucked tradition": Small, H. (1999). *Florence Nightingale: Avenging angel*. New York: St. Martin's Press, 1–19.

8. "during 1854's Crimean War"; "Queen of England with a $250,000 prize": Florence Nightingale, a nurse, spent her night rounds giving personal care to the wounded, establishing her image as the 'Lady with the Lamp.' (n.d.). Retrieved March 09, 2016, from http://www.biography.com/people/florence -nightingale-9423539#pioneering-nurse

9. "the Lady with the Lamp": Lee, Sidney, ed. (1912). Nightingale, Florence. *Dictionary of National Biography*, 1912 supplement 3. London: Smith, Elder & Co.

10. "reduced the death rate at the hospital by two-thirds": Nightingale, Florence (August 1999). *Florence Nightingale: Measuring Hospital Care Outcomes*. ISBN 0-86688-559-5. Retrieved 13 March 2010.

11. "During her tenure at Scutari": Gill, Christopher J.; Gill, Gillian C. (June 2005). Nightingale in Scutari: Her Legacy Reexamined. *Clinical Infectious Diseases* 40 (12): 1799–1805. doi:10.1086/430380. ISSN 1058-4838. PMID 15909269.

12. "By age 38": Cook, E. T. (1913). *The life of Florence Nightingale* (Vol. 1). London: Macmillan and, Limited, 237.

13. "She published a book": Nightingale, Florence (1974) [First published 1859]. Preface. In. *Notes on Nursing: What it is and what it is not.* Glasgow and London: Blackie & Son Ltd. ISBN 0-216-89974-5.

14. "consulted during America's Civil War ": Florence Nightingale and Lynn McDonald (Editor) (2010). An introduction to Vol 14. *Florence Nightingale: The Crimean War.* Wilfrid Laurier University Press. ISBN 0-88920-469-1.

15. "Even in the case of ": Taylor, F. W. (1911). *The Principles of Scientific Management.* New York: Harper & Brothers, 60, 65, 66, 85.

16. "shovel was 21 pounds": Taylor, F. W. (1911). *The Principles of Scientific Management.* New York, NY: Norton, 65–66.

17. "a fair day's pay for a fair day's work": Hutchinson, J. G. (1963). *Managing a fair day's work; an analysis of work standards in operation.* Ann Arbor: Bureau of Industrial Relations, University of Michigan, 31.

CHAPTER 14—THE UNEXPECTED INTRUDER

1. "philosopher Hans Jonas asserted that": Jonas, H. (1969). *Philosophical reflections on experimenting with human subjects.* Boston, MA: American Academy of Arts and Sciences.

2. "Dr. John Hall": Eccles, M., & Joseph, H. (1966). Shakespeare's Son-in-Law: John Hall, Man and Physician. *Shakespeare Quarterly*, 17(4), 432.

3. "translates to *shopkeeper*": Ayto, J. (2005). *Word Origins: The Hidden Histories of English Words From A to Z (Secret Histories of English Words From A to Z).* A & C Black.

4. "Hohenstaufen ruled that": Anderson, S. (2005). Making medicines: A brief history of pharmacy and pharmaceuticals. London: Pharmaceutical Press.

5. "sickness funds": Knox, R. (2008, July 3). History Of Tinkering Helps German System Endure. Retrieved March 09, 2016, from http://www.npr.org/templates /story/story.php?storyId=92189596

6. "guild memberships": Geremek, B. (2006). *The margins of society in late medieval Paris.* Cambridge: Cambridge University Press, 190.

7. "collecting boxes": Abel-Smith, B. (2013, June 5). Social security. Retrieved March 09, 2016, from http://www.britannica.com/topic/social -security-government-program

8. "to calculate the currency value of ": Ciecka. J (2008). Edmond Halley's Life Table and Its Uses. *Journal of Legal Economics*, 15(1): 65-74.

9. "'Iron' chancellor": Otto von Bismarck. (n.d.). Retrieved March 09, 2016, from http://www.history.com/topics/otto-von-bismarck

10. "welfare state": Hennock, E. P. (2007). *The origin of the welfare state in England and Germany: 1850–1914: Social policies compared*. Cambridge: Cambridge Univ. Press.

CHAPTER 15—MEDICINE'S NEW MYSTICAL FORCE

1. "When I encountered one of these": Mattern, S. (2008). *Galen and the Rhetoric of Healing* (1st ed.). Johns Hopkins University Press, 53.

2. "a newly slaughtered meat": Mattern, S. P. (2013). *The prince of medicine: Galen in the Roman Empire*. New York: Oxford University Press.

3. "The physician knows everything": *United States Naval Medical Bulletin Published for the Information of the Medical Department of the Service* (Vol. 14). (1920). Washington Government Printing Office: The Bureau of Medicine and surgery, Navy Deparment, 232.

4. "All true knowledge": Thorndike, L. (1923). *A history of magic and experimental science: During the first thirteen centuries of our era*. New York: Columbia University Press, 847.

5. "at a Spanish hospital perfecting": Gilman, D. C.; Thurston, H. T.; Colby, F. M., eds. (1905). Auenbrugger, Leopold von. *New International Encyclopedia* (1st ed.). New York: Dodd, Mead.

6. "Graduating in 1813": Simmons, J. (2002). Doctors and discoveries: Lives that created today's medicine. Boston: Houghton Mifflin, 75–79.

7. "Louis spent nearly seven years": Morabia, A. (2006). Pierre-Charles-Alexandre Louis and the evaluation of bloodletting. *Journal of the Royal Society of Medicine* 99 (3): 158–160.

8. "laid their heads upon a soft bosom": Gordon, R. (1993). *The alarming history of medicine: Amusing anecdotes from Hippocrates to heart transplants*. New York: St. Martin's Griffin, 97.

9. "Laënnec spent the next three years": Kligfield, P. (1981). Laennec and the discovery of mediate auscultation. *The American Journal of Medicine*, 70(2), 275-278.

10. "stethoscope was born": Clendening, L. (1942). *Source book of medical history* (1st ed.). New York: Harper & Brothers, 313–330.

11. "Laënnec was able to": Major, R. H. (1954). *A history of medicine*. Springfield, IL: Thomas, 661–62.

12. "therapeutics remained subordinate": Middleton W.S. (1924). A biographic history of physical diagnosis. *Ann Med Hist,* 6:426–52.

13. "average life expectancy of a 10-year-old": Diabetes History – Defeat Diabetes Foundation. (2014). Retrieved March 09, 2016, from http://www.defeatdiabetes .org/diabetes-history/

14. "Sapira directs physicians": Orient, J. M., & Sapira, J. D. (2009). *Sapira's art & science of bedside diagnosis* (4th ed.). Philadelphia: Lippincott Williams & Wilkins, 324.

15. "paradoxically be *less* likely": Is an Older, More Experienced Doctor a Better Doctor? (2005). *Annals of Internal Medicine,* 142(4). doi:10.7326/0003 -4819-142-4-200502150-00004

16. "wasn't a good enough doctor": Smith, R. (2015). David Sackett Obituary. *BMJ.* 350:h2639.

17. "180 new drugs to treat diabetes": Read More About Medicines in Development for Diabetes. (n.d.). Retrieved March 09, 2016, from http://www.phrma.org /research/medicines-development-diabetes

CHAPTER 16—TRANSCENDING LIMITATIONS

1. "The arrangements of the atoms": Schrödinger, E. (1967). *What is life?: The physical aspect of the living cell & Mind and matter*. Cambridge: University Press.

CHAPTER 17—MAN-MACHINE SYMBIOSIS

1. "every 125 flight hours": Jeffries, S. (2014). Secrets of the black box: How does MH370's flight recorder work? Retrieved March 09, 2016, from http://www.theguardian.com /world/2014/mar/31/airplane-black-box-flight-recorders-investigators

2. "Smart Tissue Autonomous Robot (STAR)": Shademan, A., Decker, R. S., Opfermann, J. D., Leonard, S., Krieger, A., & Kim, P. C. (2016). Supervised autonomous robotic soft tissue surgery. *Science Translational Medicine, 8*(337), 337. doi:10.1126/scitranslmed.aad9398

3. "For Denise Parker": Mansfield, K., & Halkon, R. (2015, November 05). Robot saves cancer patient grandmother's life. Retrieved December 26, 2016, from http://www.mirror.co.uk/news/uk-news/robot-saves-grandmothers-life-pioneering-6779392

4. "targeted nanorobotic delivery": Felfoul, O., Mohammadi, M., Taherkhani, S., Lanauze, D. D., Xu, Y. Z., Loghin, D., Martel, S. (2016). Magneto-aerotactic bacteria deliver drug-containing nanoliposomes to tumour hypoxic regions. *Nature Nanotechnology*, 11(11), 941-947. doi:10.1038/nnano.2016.137

5. "Organ Care System": Albin, A. (2010, December 06). 'Beating heart' technology could revolutionize field of heart transplantation. Retrieved December 26, 2016, from http://newsroom.ucla.edu/releases/ucla-led-study-of-beating-heart-165987

6. "3D printer to create bone fragments": Atala, A., MD. (2016). Scientists Prove Feasibility of "Printing" Replacement Tissue. Retrieved December 26, 2016, from http://bit.ly/1LsLd6v

7. "when Hurricane Katrina ravaged": Gardner, A., & Reporter, H. (2016, March 23). Electronic Medical Records Proved Their Worth in Katrina's Wake. Retrieved December 26, 2016, from http://abcnews.go.com/Health/Healthday/story?id=4506718&page=1

8. "Craig Lambert": Ehrenreich, B. (2015). 'Rise of the Robots' and 'Shadow Work'. Retrieved December 26, 2016, from http://www.nytimes.com/2015/05/17/books/review/rise-of-the-robots-and-shadow-work.html?_r=1

9. "in the service of an institutional master": Keynes, J. M. (2008). Economic Possibilities for our Grandchildren (1930). *Revisiting Keynes*, 17–26. doi:10.7551/mitpress/9780262162494.003.0002

10. "care they received lower when doctors": Ratanawongsa, N., Barton, J. L., Lyles, C. R., Wu, M., Yelin, E. H., Martinez, D., & Schillinger, D. (2016). Association between Clinician Computer Use and Communication With Patients in Safety-Net Clinics. *JAMA Internal Medicine*, 176(1), 125. doi:10.1001/jamainternmed.2015.6186

11. "43 percent of their time": Hill, R. G., Sears, L. M., & Melanson, S. W. (2013). 4000 Clicks: a productivity analysis of electronic medical records in a community hospital ED. *The American Journal of Emergency Medicine, 31*(11), 1591–1594. doi:10.1016/j.ajem.2013.06.028

12. "Most of the time devoted to": Licklider, J. C. (1960). Man-Computer Symbiosis. *IRE Transactions on Human Factors in Electronics*, HFE-1(1), 4–11.

13. "computerized diagnosis aids do not yet measure up": Semigran, H. L., Linder, J. A., Gidengil, C., & Mehrotra, A. (2015). Evaluation of symptom checkers for self-diagnosis and triage: audit study. *Bmj*, 351. doi:10.1136/bmj.h3480

CHAPTER 18—HOW WE MADE THE MODERN DOCTOR

1. "Oh! I bless the good Lord for my Boils": *Faith and Doubt of John Betjeman: An Anthology of His Religious Verse*. edited by Kevin J. Gardner, Page 192.

2. "on our DNA": Hurley, D. (2015, June 25). Grandma's Experiences Leave a Mark on Your Genes. *Discover*.

3. "I would like a doctor": Broyard, A. (1993). *Intoxicated by my illness: And other writings on life and death*. New York: Fawcett Columbine.

INDEX

PAP smears, 106
Paracelsus, 42, 165, 228
Paris Academics of Science and Medicine, 115
Parker, Denise, 238
Pascal, Blaise, 86
Pasteur, Louis, 117
Paul III (pope), 54
Pearson, Karl, 118
Pelletier, Pierre Joseph, 90
pendulum clocks, 128
Persian culture, 44–45
Pfizer Inc., 105
pharmacists and pharmacies
    development of, 201–3
    priest-physicians as pharmacists, 202
    separation of physicians and, 203
PhD (Doctor of Philosophy), 76
philosopher-physicians, 233. *See also names of*
specific philosopher-physicians
    Galen's strengthening of philosopher-phy-
        sician connection, 39–40
    Hippocrates' separation of philosopher
        and physician, 35–36
    rise of metaphysics, 90–94
    transformation into scientists, 134–35
"Philosophical Essay on Probabilities"
    (Laplace), 112
philosophy, 43, 227. *See also* Grecian culture
    and science; *names of specific philosophers*
    heart as capable of independent thought,
        144
    as required course for physicians, 75–76
    separation from psychology, 132
phlegm
    humoral theory, 32–33
    mental attitudes represented by, 33
    season associated with, 38
physical theories, 111
physicians, 135, 176. *See also* diagnosis; *names*
of specific physicians; philosopher-physicians;
priest-physicians
    acknowledging patient's faith, 261
    adapting to demands of system, 260
    compassion, 260–62
    dealing with difficult patients, 259–60

dealing with existential questions, 8–9,
    25, 252–54
delaying death, 10
discovering and naming body parts, 64
electronic documentation and, 243–44
emotions and desensitization, 175–81
empathy, 179–81
ethics, 200
experience vs. effectiveness, 221–22
explaining choices when facing terminal
    illness, 25–26
explaining reasons behind illness, 21–25
Galen's strengthening of philosopher-
    physician connection, 39–40
gray area of recommendations by, 106
healing by, 16
healing isolated diseases and parts, 9,
    69–70, 197, 231, *233*
high expectations regarding, 200–201,
    211, 253
Hippocrates' separation of priest/
    philosopher and, 34–36
inclination to resign from caring for dying
    patients, 183–84
joining network of sciences, 112
lack of access to primary care physicians,
    237
listening, 255–56, 258
as mechanics, 71
mindfulness, 258–59
modern role of, 255–56
narrative-based engagement, 174–76,
    182, 255–56
as nature's assistant, 34–35, 42
personal beliefs of, 16
philosophy as required course for, 75–76
prayer and, 16
priests vs., 17
role of, 8–9, 24
shadow work, 243–45, 259
slowing down process of care, 258–59
specialization, 254–56
statistics as vital part of training, 119
tradition of perfecting theories and
    philosophies of predecessors, 58, 65

ABOUT THE AUTHOR

Rajeev Kurapati, MD, practices Hospital Medicine in Northern Kentucky. He holds an MBA from the University of Missouri and writes on health, wellness, and culture. His first book, *Unbound Intelligence*, won the 2014 National Indie Excellence Award and was a finalist in the USA Best Book Awards. Born and raised in India, he now resides in Cincinnati, Ohio, with his family.